Urology and the Primary Care Practitioner

Larry I. Lipshultz, MD
Editor
Professor of Urology
Scott Department of Urology
Baylor College of Medicine
Houston, Texas

Isaac Kleinman, MD
Associate Editor and Consultant
Associate Professor of Family Medicine
Baylor College of Medicine
Houston, Texas

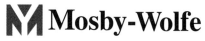 **Mosby-Wolfe**

MEDICAL COMMUNICATIONS

London   Baltimore   Bogota   Boston   Buenos Aires   Caracas   Carlsbad   Chicago   Madrid   Mexico City   Milan
Naples   New York   Philadelphia   St. Louis   Singapore   Sydney   Tokyo   Toronto   Wiesbaden

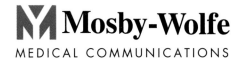

Mosby-Wolfe

MEDICAL COMMUNICATIONS

**A Times Mirror
International Publisher**

Publisher:	David K. Marshall
Senior Editor:	Beth Adams
Editorial Coordinator:	Jennifer Yarrish
Project Manager:	Chris Baumle
Production Editor:	David Orzechowski
Design Manager:	Nancy McDonald
Manufacturing Supervisor:	Bill Winneberger
Illustration:	Jan Redden

Copyright © 1995 Times Mirror International Publishers Limited

Published in 1995 by Mosby-Wolfe Medical Communications, a division of Times Mirror International Publishers Limited

Printed by Rand McNally

ISBN 0–7234–2482–9

For full details of all Times Mirror International Publishers Limited titles, please write to Times Mirror International Publishers Limited, Lynton House, 7–12 Tavistock Square, London WC1H 9LB, England.

A CIP catalogue record of this book is available from the British Library.

Preface

This book is written primarily for family practitioners and other primary care physicians, but will also be helpful to anyone wishing to review the essentials of diagnosis and treatment of commonly seen urologic diseases. The content of this book represents the consensus of a sizable group of physicians with broad clinical experience. All contributors are members of the Scott Department of Urology and have worked together at the Baylor-Affiliated Hospitals of the Texas Medical Center. They were chosen for their expertise in the various specialized areas of urology and invited to address these areas in their respective chapters.

We wish to express our gratitude to the contributors for their diligent work, comprehensive yet concise coverage of their topics, and their identification of important urologic problems that would be of special interest to the primary care physician. We would also like to thank our in-house editor, Carolyn Schum, M.A., for her countless hours of work in seeing this book to its completion.

Larry I. Lipshultz, MD
Editor

Isaac Kleinman, MD
Associate Editor and Consultant

Contributors

**From the Scott Department of Urology
Baylor College of Medicine
Houston, Texas**

Timothy B. Boone, MD, PhD
Michael Coburn, MD
Irving J. Fishman, MD
Angelo E. Gousse, MD
John A. Greer, MD
Donald P. Griffith, MD
Tayfun Gürpinar, MD
John R. Harding, MD
John L. Hinson, MD
Seth P. Lerner, MD
Ronald A. Morton, Jr., MD
David R. Roth, MD
Kevin M. Slawin, MD
Richard W. Sutherland, MD
Mark Sutton, MD

Contents

Introduction

Larry I. Lipshultz, MD
Isaac Kleinman, MD

The last 5 years have brought a significant change in the interaction of patients, their family care physicians, and surgical specialists. Once able to bypass the primary care physician and go directly to a provider of specialized medical care, patients now find themselves obliged by the newer insurance programs to seek initial evaluation by their family doctors (primary care physicians/PCP) before referral to a specialist. As a consequence, the PCP is under increased pressure to evaluate patients with a myriad of systemic complaints rapidly and cost-effectively, to treat them when appropriate, and to refer them to other physicians only when necessary.

Because of the large number and wide variety of symptoms and underlying pathological conditions that may be traced to the genitourinary system, the PCP will see many patients whose problems are of genitourinary origin. It is the purpose of this text is to identify the most common urologic problems, to address the appropriateness and correct interpretation of specific diagnostic tests, and to help the PCP determine when specialized urologic care is most appropriate.

The text focuses initially on the physical examination of patients reporting urinary tract problems and then progresses to the most common of the urologic disorders and the signs and symptoms most often associated with them. Specific urologic problems are then addressed, the emphasis being on initial diagnosis and first-line therapy. Topics, such as recurrent urinary tract infections in both the male and the female and female urinary tract incontinence are addressed with special attention to the specific types of incontinence most commonly identified. Complaints associated with the prostate gland are certainly some of the most common complaints of male patients, and, consequently, one section is devoted to prostate cancer. It includes a review of most common signs and symptoms and describes the appropriate work-up and subsequent staging and treatment of prostate cancer. Another section is devoted to evaluation of nonmalignant diseases of the prostate. With patients now less reticent to discuss problems once considered "too personal and embarrassing," we have addressed two of the more common complaints reported by patients to their PCP, erectile dysfunction and infertility. A special chapter discusses the evaluation of infants with the undescended testes, since this is the congenital abnormality of the genitourinary tract most commonly encountered by the PCP. Finally, the text concludes with a review of urologic emergencies and emphasizes emergency procedures that the PCP may have to perform.

It is hoped that the PCP reading this text will achieve a better understanding of current methods for diagnosing urologic complaints and will gain insight into when first-line therapy should be introduced and when referral to the urologic specialist is appropriate and necessary. A productive partnership between the PCP and the medical or surgical specialist—in this case, the urologist—is the best mechanism by which patients operating under the medical guidelines of the 1990s can benefit from the medical system. Only when the patient, the PCP, and the specialist work as a cohesive team is the patient assured optimal medical care.

1

Physical Examination of the External Male Genitalia

Examination of the external male genitalia is unique when compared with examination of other organ systems or regional examinations because the male genitalia are so easily inspected and palpated. However, many physicians perform only a rudimentary examination of the genitalia because of a lack of familiarity with the examination or their own personal reluctance to perform the examination. This is, indeed, unfortunate, as many of the most common malignancies affecting the male genitalia can be detected by physical examination alone. Testicular cancer, the most common type of malignant tumor in men aged 20 to 35 years, is easily palpated on examination. Prostate cancer, the malignancy most frequently diagnosed in men and second only to lung cancer as a cause of cancer death, can also frequently be palpated.

Consequently, the need for a thorough understanding of and familiarity with examination of the male external genitalia can be appreciated. Outlined here is a systematic approach to this examination as well as a basic fund of knowledge that can be enhanced by continued experience. Patients with certain identifiable abnormalities and disorders should be referred to a specialist in urology.

INFRAPUBIC REGION

Examination of the genitalia may be performed with the patient in either an erect or a supine position. The inspection begins within the infrapubic region. The distribution of pubic hair should be noted. In adolescents, documentation of the appropriate Tanner stage of genital development is indicated. Obvious abnormal skin lesions should be noted. These may include nevi, venereal warts, rashes, or scabies. A brief examination above the pubic bone through inspection, percussion, and palpation can assist in detection of a distended bladder, which indicates inadequate emptying.

PENIS

Examination of the penis logically occurs next. The penile shaft is made of two paired erectile bodies known as the corpora cavernosa, which are located dorsolaterally. A smaller, single erectile body, the corpus spongiosum, is located ventrally at the midline and surrounds the urethra. The distal extent of the penis is covered by a cone-shaped tissue known as the glans penis. The proximal rolled edge of the glans penis is known as the corona. Presence or absence of a foreskin, or prepuce, should be noted. In adults, retraction of the foreskin proximally to expose the inner preputial mucosal surface and the glans penis should be easily performed. Any resistance to retraction may be indicative of acute or chronic inflammation or scarring.

Phimosis is the inability to retract the foreskin proximally because of narrowing of the foreskin surface or preputial scarring. Pliability of the foreskin is variable in children until approximately five years of age, when the foreskin usually becomes easily retractable, as in adults. Any attempt to forcibly retract the foreskin in a child is ill-advised, as iatrogenic pain, bleeding, and subsequent scarring may result. *Paraphimosis* is the inability to return the foreskin distally over the glans penis after it has been retracted. In children, this is usually secondary to self-exploration or the mother's efforts at hygiene. In adults, this pathology is frequently iatrogenic and may develop in a hospital setting if the foreskin is retracted for cleansing or instrumentation and not returned over the glans penis. Subsequent constriction and swelling of the shaft and glans in a distal direction may compromise vascularity. A dorsal slit of the foreskin or circumcision may be necessary to resolve this emergent situation. However, if paraphimosis is detected early, simple manipulation and reduction of the foreskin may remedy the situation (see the chapter on Urologic Emergencies).

After inspection of the foreskin and glans penis, the urethral meatus is examined. The urethral opening should be solitary and located at the distal tip of the glans penis. Hypospadias is an aberrant opening proximal and ventral to the standard meatal opening. Epispadias is a dorsally located meatal opening. Gentle retraction of the meatus by placing each thumb laterally to the meatus while the index fingers are placed on the lateral coronal edge may reveal proximal urethral lesions (e.g., warts) or proximal strictures. This maneuver is especially important in young men who have concerns regarding a sexually transmitted disease. Any discharge from the meatus should be cultured to exclude *Neisseria gonorrhoeae* and *Chlamydia trachomatis*.

After examination of the distal penis, the penile shaft is inspected and palpated. Any curvatures or irregularities of the skin and erectile bodies should be noted. Chordee, a ventral penile curvature, is commonly associated with hypospadias. In infants with hypospadias, bilateral compression with the index fingers lateral to the base of the penis may assist in assessing the extent of curvature. This maneuver stretches the penile skin over the corporeal bodies and may simulate an erection; the maneuver should be used as a guide and not as a definitive diagnosis of chordee.

Palpation of the corpus cavernosum and corpus spongiosum is especially important in adults. Induration or plaques within the corpus cavernosum may indicate Peyronie's disease. Ventral induration or a mass within the urethra suggests internal disease; malignancy or inflammation must be excluded. "Milking of the urethra," by compressing it from a proximal position to a distal position, should be performed to exclude a urethral discharge. At the ventral base of the penis in children, the penoscrotal junction should be examined. Any penoscrotal fusion should be evaluated by a pediatric urologist.

SCROTUM

As with the infrapubic region and penis, any abnormal skin lesions should be noted. The scrotal skin normally is rugose and very pliable. Thickened, indurated, or nonpliable skin suggests a pathologic skin process. However, edema from various systemic sources, such as congestive heart failure or liver failure, may result in scrotal swelling without pathology within the skin itself. The proximity of the scrotum to the body varies, depending on body habitus and resting tone of the underlying dartos musculature. The scrotal sac is divided into two separate compartments by a midline septum. Within each compartment, or hemiscrotum, lies a testicle, epididymis, and spermatic cord (Fig. 1–1). These structures should be freely mobile within each hemiscrotum.

Several benign scrotal skin conditions occur frequently and deserve mention in a discussion of the scrotal examination. Infection of the crural folds, scrotum, and prepuce with *Candida albicans* is quite common. This infection typically occurs in association with diabetes mellitus, use of antibiotics, immunosuppression, and when genital skin is made more hospitable to the organism with sweat retention and moisture. The hallmark of cutaneous candidiases is bright-red inflammation. Inflammation spreads in a radial fashion and does not have sharp, distinct borders at the edge of involved skin. Small pustules can often be seen overlying the red plaque. The degree of associated pruritus varies greatly. Tinea cruris is also a common fungal infection of the genital area. Classically, lesions are dusky, red-brown patches seen on the inner thighs. The most active region of inflammation has a thin, red ring at the periphery. This accounts

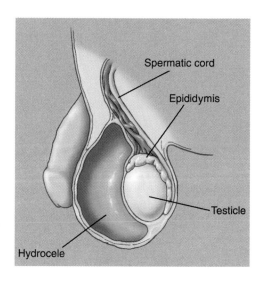

FIG. 1–1.

Schematic representation of the testicle, epididymis, spermatic cord, and a hydrocele.

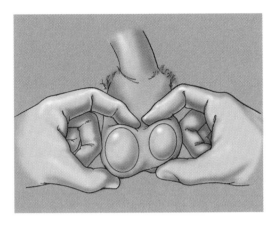

FIG. 1–2.

Simultaneous comparison of testicular size demonstrating left testicular atrophy.

for the colloquial term "ringworm." Both candidiasis and tinea cruris can be treated with most common antifungal medications, such as naftifine hydrochloride and imidazoles, although tinea cruris responds poorly to nystatin.

Skin lesions unrelated to infectious etiologies also are common. Epidermoid cysts can occur throughout the body but may be especially striking when found in the scrotal skin. These cysts are white to skin colored, firm, and 1 to 2 centimeters in diameter. They are typically asymptomatic and can be multiple. No specific treatment is required unless a patient demands treatment for cosmetic reasons. Angiokeratomas also are common as well as benign. These scrotal lesions, which are found in 20% of adult men, are very small (1 to 2 millimeters) papular hemangiomas that are red to violet in color. Typically, multiple lesions are scattered throughout the surface of the scrotum. These lesions are usually asymptomatic and require no treatment. However, if bleeding occurs, electrocautery and laser treatment can be used.

Testicle

The testicle should be gently palpated between the thumb and the index and middle fingers. The size, shape, and consistency of the testicle should be noted. The testicle is ovoid in shape, measuring 4 centimeters or more longitudinally and 2.5 centimeters or more transversely. In consistency, the testicles should be firm and slightly rubbery. The testicles should be symmetric in shape, size, and consistency (Fig. 1–2). Documenting size is especially important in adolescents and infertile men. Commercially available orchidometers (ASSI, Westbury, NY) can be used to document testicular volumes for comparison. The testicle should have a smooth, regular surface and lie in a dependent position in the scrotum. If testicles are not palpable in the scrotum, a more proximal examination of the inguinal canal should ensue to exclude cryptorchidism. Irregularities of the testicular surface or a mass within the testicle should be promptly referred to the urologist to rule out a possible tumor.

Difficulty in palpating a testicle in an enlarged hemiscrotum may be secondary to a hydrocele. The testicle is covered by a visceral and parietal extension of the peritoneum known as the tunica vaginalis. Fluid accumulation between these layers results in a hydrocele (Fig. 1–1). Transillumination in a darkened room using a penlight or similar light source is helpful in distinguishing between a fluid-filled structure (positive transillumination) and a solid mass. On occasion, auscultation of scrotal enlargement may reveal peristaltic sounds that confirm a hernia extruding into the scrotum.

Epididymis

Examination of the epididymis is intimately associated with the testicular examination because the epididymis typically lies on the superior and posterior surface of the testicle. The epididymides are also symmetric and allow for direct comparison of both sides. The epididymis is softer in consistency than the testicle and is felt as a posterior elevated ridge. Examination of the epididymis should be done very gently because it may be extremely sensitive.

Anatomically, the epididymis can be divided into three segments: the caput (head), corpus (body), and cauda (tail). Each corresponds with the superior, middle, and inferior portions, respectively. Enlargement or tenderness of the epididymis typically is due to inflammation (epididymitis). Cystic lesions of the epididymis, such as a spermatocele, allow the transmission of light and will consequently transilluminate.

Spermatic Cord

After examination of the epididymis is complete, the spermatic cord is palpated. If the patient is supine, having him stand upright is helpful for this portion of the examination. Typically, the examination starts midway between the external ring and testicle. Identification of the vas deferens should be easily accomplished. The vas deferens has a characteristic cord-like shape and consistency. Although much more flexible and slightly larger in diameter, the vas deferens feels similar to the wire found in a coat hanger. If the vas deferens cannot be palpated, further special studies are indicated.

Other cord structures are less distinct. Classically, a varicocele has been described as similar in appearance and feel to a bag of worms. Certainly, a grossly enlarged and tortuous spermatic vein gives such an impression. However, in most instances, a varicocele is more subtle. For clearest identification of a varicocele, one cord is grasped in each hand separately between the thumb and first two fingers (Fig. 1–3*A*). After the cords are isolated, any dilated vascular structures can be noted (Fig. 1–3*B*). The patient is then asked to perform a Valsalva maneuver. An increase in the size suggests a small varicocele. An active cremasteric reflex may make the examination less precise. Although more frequently seen on the left, varicoceles they can occur bilaterally.

Further palpation of the cord should be performed. Rubbery, fleshy masses of the cord may indicate a lipoma or, rarely, a liposarcoma. Cystic masses of the cord that transilluminate most commonly are loculated hydroceles of the cord. If the patient is asymptomatic, these findings usually require no specific intervention. If the diagnosis is unclear, the patient should be referred to a urologist.

The scrotal evaluation is complete after examination for an inguinal hernia. The index finger is passed over the scrotal skin and spermatic cord proximally toward the external inguinal ring (Fig. 1–4). Once the external ring is palpated, the patient is asked to cough or perform a Valsalva maneuver. A palpable impulse or bulge indicates an inguinal hernia.

In summary, during a scrotal examination, the testicle; epididymis; spermatic cord; and, lastly, the external inguinal ring are palpated systematically. Testicular masses are usually malignant and must be fully evaluated. Masses of

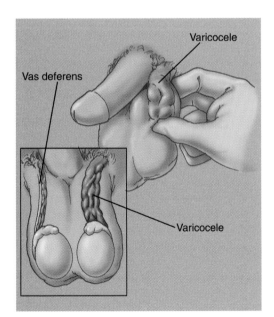

FIG. 1–3.

A, Palpation of the spermatic cords. **B,** Schematic representation of the vas deferens and spermatic vessels demonstrating a left varicocele.

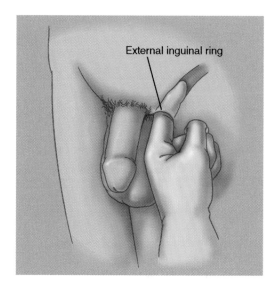

External inguinal ring

FIG. 1–4.

Palpation of the external inguinal canal to examine for an inguinal hernia.

the epididymis and spermatic cord typically are benign but nevertheless require a definitive diagnosis. Examination of the male genitalia should include instruction on testicular self-examination in the post-pubertal age group. Printed instructions are available from a number of sources. Acute scrotal pain and emergencies are addressed in another chapter.

PROSTATE

Although the prostate is not an external organ, a complete examination of the male genitalia involves a rectal examination to palpate the prostate. The American Foundation for Urologic Disease recommends that all men older than 50 years of age have an annual rectal examination to examine the prostate and a serum prostate-specific antigen (PSA) assay. In Blacks as well as in men with a family history of prostate cancer, the examination should be done on a yearly basis beginning at age 40. Although concern has been raised about obtaining a PSA after a digital prostate examination because of potential exam-related serum increases, recent studies have failed to demonstrate a significant elevation in PSA after a simple digital examination. Thus, a PSA level can be drawn *after* a prostate examination, if convenient.

In young males, the prostate typically is 3.5 centimeters transversely by 2.5 centimeters longitudinally and weighs 18 to 20 grams. The gland has been described as being similar to a chestnut in configuration. An enlarged prostate is common after the age of 50; thus, normal dimensions vary significantly with age. A normal prostate has a consistency similar to the thenar eminence when the thumb opposes the little finger.

The patient may be positioned in several ways to allow for easy digital access to the prostate. A lateral decubitus position, with the legs flexed at the hip and knees towards the chest, allows comfortable access. Another option that facilitates access is to have the patient stand with his back toward the physician and bend 90° at the waist with his elbows on the examining table (Fig. 1–5A). After the examining hand is covered with a disposable glove, a generous amount of water-soluble lubricant is placed over the examining finger. The

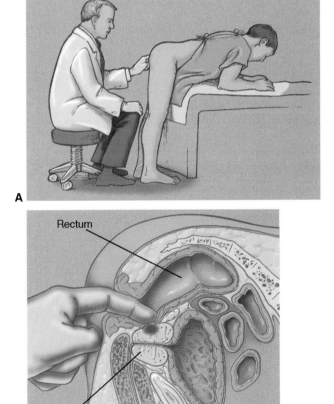

FIG. 1–5.

A, Demonstration of a rectal examination in the standing position. **B,** Palpation of a prostatic nodule.

buttocks are separated, and the anus is inspected for pathology. The gloved index finger is then gently placed at the anal orifice, where gentle pressure is applied. This maneuver allows for relaxation of the anal sphincter and results in a more comfortable examination for the patient as anal tone is assessed. After the anal sphincter has relaxed, the lubricated index finger is passed into the rectal vault over the prostate. The examining finger should be inserted far enough to allow digital examination of the entire posterior surface of the prostate.

Examination typically begins at the apex (closest to the anal sphincter) and proceeds to the base. A sweeping motion of the finger allows appreciation of the lateral lobes and central sulcus. Abnormalities should be described as *right* or *left* as well as *apical, base, midline,* or *lateral.* The seminal vesicles arise from the base of the prostate and are not normally palpable. During palpation of the prostate, an estimation of size is obtained. Although urologists tend to measure size in terms of grams or on a scale of 0 to 4, it is better to note the gland size in centimeters in the transverse and longitudinal planes. In addition to size, the prostate should be assessed for symmetry. Asymmetry should be noted, and any irregularity or induration should raise suspicion of malignancy or inflammation or infection (Fig. 1–5*B*). An acutely inflamed prostate may feel boggy (i.e., unusually soft) and be tender. Fluctuance suggests the presence of an abscess. Vigorous massage of an acutely inflamed prostate should be avoided.

Prior to removal of the examining finger, a circumferential sweep of the rectal vault should be completed to exclude rectal pathology. After the examination, the patient should be offered tissues to remove any excess lubricant. After completion of the prostate examination, penile discharge or expressed prostatic secretions should be examined microscopically.

URINALYSIS

Urinalysis is an important part of the urologic examination. A urine specimen should be obtained at midstream, using a "clean-catch" method (Box 1–1 on page 12). The color of the urine is noted (Table 1–1). Noncentrifuged urine is examined with a dipstick colorimetric chemical assay for urine pH, glucose, protein, free hemoglobin, ketones, bilirubin, urobilinogen, nitrites, and leukocyte esterase. A sample of the urine is then centrifuged for 3 to 5 minutes at approximately 2,500 rpm. The supernatant is discarded, and the remaining sediment is mixed with the small amount of urine left in the tube. Microscopic examination is then performed under low and high power (Table 1–2). The number of red blood cells, white blood cells, budding yeast, bacteria, crystals, and/or casts per high-power microscopic field (HPF) are observed and quantified. A urine culture is obtained if infection is suggested by the urinalysis or clinical presentation. A dipstick test that is positive for *both* nitrites and leuko-

TABLE 1–1.

Common Causes of Abnormal Urine Color

| Color | Etiology | | |
	Disease	Drugs	Miscellaneous
None	Diabetes mellitus	Ethyl alcohol	Overhydration
	Diabetes insipidus	Diuretics	
Yellow-orange		Tetracycline	Dehydration
		Flutamide	
		Pyridium	
		Azo-Gantrisin®	
		(Roche Laboratories)	
		Sulfasalazine	
		Vitamin B	
Milky white	Urinary tract infection/pyuria		
	Chyluria		
Blue-green	*Pseudomonas* urinary tract infection	Methylene blue	
		Urised	
		Indigo carmine	
		Doan's Pills®	
		(Ciba Consumer)	
		Clorets	
		Elavil®	
		(Stuart Pharmaceuticals)	
Red-brown	Hematuria	Rifampin	Beets
	Hemolytic anemia	Ex-Lax®	Blackberries
	Hemoglobinuria	(Sandoz Consumer)	Rhubarb
	Myoglobinuria	Phenolphthalein	
	Lead poisoning	Phenothiazines	
	Mercury poisoning	Nitrofurantoin	
	Porphyria	Doxorubicin	
Brown-black	Fecaluria	Metronidazole	Fava beans
	Methemoglobinuria	Methyldopa	Aloe
	Melaninuria	Methocarbamol	

BOX 1–1.

Instructions for Obtaining a "Clean Catch" Midstream Urine Specimen

It is important to catch your urine specimen as "cleanly" as possible. Otherwise, it may pick up germs from the skin and lead the laboratory to report signs of infection in the urine when there really is none. Follow these steps carefully in collecting your urine specimen:

Females

1. Avoid contacting the inside of the specimen container or the inside of its lid with any part of your body.
2. With one hand, spread the lips of the genital area and keep them apart.
3. Using your free hand, wipe the area once or twice from front to back using the cotton ball or towelette provided by the nurse.
4. Start to urinate into the toilet
5. Then urinate into the container until it is half full.
6. Finish urinating into the toilet.
7. Carefully cap the specimen container.

Males

1. Avoid contacting the inside of the specimen container or the inside of its lid with any part of your body.
2. With one hand, pull back your foreskin (if uncircumcised) and hold it back.
3. With your free hand, wipe off the end of the penis with the cotton balls or towelette provided by the nurse.
4. Start to urinate into the toilet.
5. Then urinate into the container until it is half full.
6. Finish urinating into the toilet.
7. Carefully cap the specimen container.

TABLE 1–2.
Normal Urinalysis Values

Specific gravity	1.008 to 1.020
pH	4.5 to 8.0
Heme	Negative
Glucose	Negative
Ketones	Negative
Protein	Negative
Bilirubin	Negative
Leukocyte esterase	Negative
Nitrites	Negative
Red blood cells	0 to 3/HPF
White blood cells	0 to 3/HPF
Bacteria	0 to 3/HPF (spun)

cyte esterase strongly suggests a urinary tract infection, as does a microscopic examination of *centrifuged* urine with 4 to 5 bacteria/HPF.

CONCLUSION

In summary, examination of the male genitalia is an essential component of any comprehensive physical examination and is mandatory in any male with urologic symptoms. Not only should this examination be completed by the physician, but a monthly testicular self-examination is advised in men 20 to 35 years of age (Fig. 1–6). A yearly digital rectal examination should also be performed by the family practitioner or urologist in men aged 50 years or older and at age 40 and older in Black men and those with a family history of prostate cancer.

The goal of any physical examination is to detect physical abnormalities in asymptomatic patients and to localize pathology in symptomatic patients. Examination of the male external genitalia uniquely allows both.

Regular (monthly) self-examination of your testicles is important because (1) testicular cancers tend to be cancers of young men and (2) when found early, they are usually curable. The examination is uncomplicated and only takes a minute.

The testicle in the scrotum feels like a small, firm, hard-boiled egg. On its back surface and top lies the epididymis, which can be separately felt as a ridge running up the backside of the testicle. The epididymis has two parts, the body and the tail, which can sometimes be felt separately. Attached to the upper pole of the testicle and running up into the groin is the spermatic cord. It is made up of muscle fibers, blood vessels, and the vas deferens. It has a slightly spongy feel, except for the vas deferens, which feels rod-like and firm. It has been described as feeling like a "rod of spaghetti."

First, look at the entire scrotum and the adjacent skin areas and note any rashes, sores, or bumps. Second, feel the scrotum and its contents carefully. Once you have done this a few times, the feel of the normal testicle, epididymis, and spermatic cord will be familiar, and any abnormality will "jump out" at you. Anything you see or feel that was not present on earlier examinations should be brought to the attention of your doctor.

It may be helpful to do this examination once in your doctor's office so that he can answer any questions you may have about what you are feeling.

FIG. 1–6.

Scrotal and testicular self-examination.

SUGGESTED READING

Bates B: *A Guide to Physical Examination and History Taking,* ed 6, Philadelphia, JB Lippincott, 1995, pp 361–375, 417–425.

DeGowin RC: *DeGowin and DeGowin's Diagnostic Examination,* ed 6, New York, MacMillan, 1994, pp 567–597.

Lowe FC, Brendler CB: Evaluation of the urologic patient, in Walsh PC and others (eds): *Campbell's Urology,* ed 6, Philadelphia, WB Saunders, 1992, pp 307–331.

Raymond JR, Yarger WE: Abnormal urine color: differential diagnosis, *Southern Med J* 81:837–841, 1988.

Van Arsdalen KN: Signs and symptoms: the initial examination, in Hanno PM, Wein AJ (eds): *Clinical Manual of Urology,* ed 2. New York, McGraw-Hill, 1994, pp 53–88.

Wyker AW: Standard diagnostic consideration, in Gillenwater JY and others (eds): *Adult and Pediatric Urology,* ed 2. St. Louis, Mosby–Year Book, 1991, pp 63–77.

2

Common Urologic Symptoms and Physical Findings: Differential Diagnosis

A discussion of the symptoms of urologic disease must include a variety of topics, ranging from voiding symptoms that are typical of urinary infection or bladder outlet obstruction, to subtle physical abnormalities that allow the physician to distinguish between acute scrotal processes, to signs of florid sepsis (such as those associated with obstruction with infection of the upper urinary tracts). Following is a discussion of the most frequent signs and symptoms of common or important urologic diseases, with emphasis on differential diagnosis. The concluding paragraphs discuss miscellaneous genital complaints.

An important principle of differential diagnosis in urology, as in most areas of medicine, is that various disease entities may lead to similar signs and symptoms. A frequently encountered example is the presence of irritative voiding symptoms, which may result from such diverse entities as urinary infection, bladder outlet obstruction with resultant detrusor instability, neurogenic bladder dysfunction, or urothelial malignancy. The history and physical examination often give important clues regarding the differential diagnosis, but additional testing may be required to establish a definitive diagnosis.

PAIN AND MASS OF UROLOGIC ORIGIN

Pain is a common symptom of many well-recognized and important urologic disease processes, such as acute renal or ureteral colic, testicular torsion, urinary retention, and certain forms of urologic trauma. In contrast, many urologic conditions of equal seriousness typically present without pain; among them are testicular tumor; early stages of renal, bladder, and prostate cancer; and the more gradual progressive forms of obstructive uropathy. It is important to recognize the significance of pain related to the urogenital system and appreciate the limitations of its diagnostic usefulness. As with any type of pain, urologic pain must be characterized by anatomic site, pattern of radiation, severity, onset, alleviating or exacerbating factors, and quality, as the patient would describe it in a clinical evaluation.

Abdominal Pain

Patients are often referred for urologic evaluation after complaining of abdominal, flank, or back pain. Excluding a urologic etiology of abdominal pain may require no more than a careful history and physical examination or may require more sophisticated testing.

As noted earlier, pain related to renal disease may result from several causes. Renal or ureteral calculi cause pain when they cause obstruction with resultant hydronephrosis. Increased pressure within the collecting system and distension of the renal capsule result in painful stimuli via visceral afferent sensory fibers. Calculi may be present in the collecting system and reach considerable size without causing pain if no obstruction is present or if obstruction progresses gradually over a prolonged time frame. This is often seen with staghorn calculi due to chronic urinary infection with urea-splitting organisms. Similarly, the disappearance of pain during documented passage of a ureteral calculus should never be presumed to indicate that the stone has passed and obstruction relieved. Over time, the obstructed renal unit accommodates to the obstructed state by the processes of pyelovenous and pyelolymphatic backflow and forniceal extravasation along with decreased urine production, resulting in decreasing pressure within the collecting system and decreased pain. If the physician fails to reassess the urinary tract radiographically, silent obstruction may persist and ultimately result in destruction of the renal unit.

Renal pain may also result from infection, acute pyelonephritis, or renal or perinephric abscess; papillary necrosis can also cause significant pain. Renal ischemia may cause pain, especially if acute in onset, as in renal arterial occlusion from arterial embolus, atherosclerotic disease, or arterial intimal disruption from deceleration trauma. Blunt trauma to the kidney causes pain from injury to the soft tissues of the flank, subcapsular hematoma, renal parenchymal injury, adjacent visceral organs, or hemoperitoneum.

Pain of renal origin is generally noted in the area of the costovertebral angle or more diffusely in the flank or upper abdominal quadrants. As calculi travel down the ureter, the symptomatology changes with the location of the stone. Stones at the ureteropelvic junction or in the upper ureter tend to produce pain in the costo-vertebral angle (CVA) region or lateral flank. In the mid-ureter, stones cause pain more caudally in the lateral abdomen. When stones are in the lower ureter, pain is often experienced in the lower quadrants; when they reach the most distal ureter or ureterovesical junction, pain may be referred to the ipsilateral testicle or the penis, or the complaint may be largely of irritative voiding symptoms due to trigonal edema and inflammation.

Lower abdominal pain may be due to urologic causes, for example, urinary retention, bladder irritation (as from infection, presence of a foreign body, or such inflammatory processes as interstitial cystitis), or trauma.

Abdominal pain of nonurologic cause may mimic that of renal origin. Common nonurologic causes of abdominal pain that may be confused with pain of urologic origin include cholelithiasis or cholecystitis, diverticulosis or diverticulitis, retroperitoneal or psoas abscess, and intraabdominal neoplasm. Combined urologic and neoplastic problems may be seen in patients with infiltrative retroperitoneal neoplasms (lymphoma or a tumor that has metastasized to the retroperitoneum), which also cause extrinsic ureteral obstruction. Back pain of musculoskeletal origin and neurologic pain from thoracolumbar disk disease may be easily confused with pain of renal origin and often prompt urologic referral.

Genital Pain and Mass

Scrotal Pain

Assessment of both acute scrotal pain and a mass effect is among the more challenging areas of urologic differential diagnosis. For example, distinguishing between acute testicular torsion and epididymitis is critical and has an immediate effect on management decisions. The differential diagnosis of common forms of scrotal pathology with the salient classic features of presentation is reviewed in the following discussion.

Testicular torsion is the most urgent scrotal condition for which accurate diagnosis and prompt attention are critical, as the timing of treatment determines the chances of testicular salvage. Onset of pain is most often abrupt and may be (but is not necessarily) associated with physical activity. Pain is usually substantial from the initial hours to early days of untreated torsion, after which there is often some decrease in the intensity of pain as infarction progresses and sensation from the involved testicle is lost. After several days, the pain often reaches another crescendo as edema and inflammation in the surrounding tunica and scrotal wall progress to an indurated, tender, painful scrotal phlegmon. If untreated, this progresses to liquefactive necrosis and formation of an abscess or to gradual atrophy.

Epididymitis usually causes pain that is more gradual in onset, and, in the early stages of presentation, is usually localized to the posterolateral region of the scrotal contents. In younger men, there is often a history of potential exposure to venereal disease or concomitant symptoms of urethritis may be present. In patients younger than 35 years of age, the most common causative agent for epididymitis is *Chlamydia trachomatis,* while enteric bacteria (e.g., *Escherichia coli, Klebsiella* sp., and *Enterococcus*) are most common in patients older than 35 years of age. In the latter group, and especially in men older than 50 years of age, symptoms of bladder outlet obstruction may coexist with epididymitis, as the pathophysiology is often related to impaired bladder emptying and resultant urinary infection that ascends to the epididymis. It is important to exclude urinary retention by palpation and percussion of the bladder or by analysis of post-void residual urine obtained by catheter or by ultrasonographic measurement.

With more severe forms of epididymitis, such hallmarks as localized epididymal induration and tenderness may be lost, and physical findings may be similar to those of late torsion. In this setting, further imaging to assess testicular perfusion or surgical exploration may be appropriate. After resolution of the infectious process, evaluation may include flow rate determination, retrograde urethrography, or cystoscopy.

Other physical findings on scrotal examination indicative of infectious or inflammatory disease may include erythema, scrotal wall fixation, fluctuance, crepitus, or purulent drainage. Advanced cases of epididymoorchitis may lead to abscess formation. Primary infection of the scrotal wall or perineal soft tissues, such as Fournier's gangrene, may be accompanied by fever, signs of sepsis, and the physical findings noted above. Immediate urologic consultation and rapid institution of medical and surgical therapy are essential, as these conditions may progress rapidly.

Testicular tumor classically presents as a painless mass within the testicle. In fact, 95% of intratesticular masses represent malignant testicular neoplasms, while the vast majority of extratesticular masses are benign. If there is any doubt regarding whether a mass is within or outside the testicle, scrotal ultrasonography and urologic consultation should be obtained.

Incarcerated inguinal hernias may present as scrotal masses, and the physician can usually appreciate the thickening at the scrotal neck, which represents the hernia sac descending from the groin into the scrotum. If intestine has herniated into the scrotum, bowel sounds may be audible by auscultation. The hernia defect is often palpable on careful groin examination, and it may be possible to reduce the hernia with the patient in a supine and relaxed position.

Other benign scrotal masses include hydrocele, spermatocele, and varicocele. Hydroceles can be painful if large or infected; they can be appreciated as fluid within the potential space between the parietal and visceral tunica vaginalis by palpating the mass and by transillumination. It is important to keep in mind that 10% to 15% of testicular neoplasms may have a concomitant reactive or malignant hydrocele, and scrotal ultrasonography should also be performed if there is any doubt regarding the normal state of the testicle in the presence of surrounding fluid.

A spermatocele is a cystic dilatation of the efferent ductules as they exit the testicles; thus, the fluid contains sperm. These cystic masses are palpable near the upper pole of the testicle (near the junction with the caput epididymis); usually are not tender; and, like benign hydroceles, should be surgically corrected if they cause such troublesome local symptoms as heaviness, discomfort, or inconvenience because of their large size.

A varicocele is a dilatation of the pampiniform plexus of veins resulting from incompetence of the venous valves of the internal spermatic venous system. Grossly, a large varicocele may demonstrate the typical bag-of-worms appearance of the multiple, dilated venous channels within the scrotum. Smaller varicoceles may be palpable when the patient performs the Valsalva maneuver while standing. Varicoceles are most common on the left side because of the asymmetry of the venous anatomy. If present solely on the right, if they remain dilated while the patient assumes the supine position, or if they occur abruptly or enlarge rapidly, the physician should be suspicious of a retroperitoneal or renal mass causing either vena caval obstruction or intraabdominal obstruction of the internal spermatic vein. Careful abdominal examination followed by appropriate imaging studies should be performed.

Penile and Urethral Pain

Penile angulation and pain may result from Peyronie's disease, which is caused by fibrosis of the tunica albuginea of the corpus cavernosa and manifests as palpable plaques along the penile shaft. Penile pain may also result from vascular compromise or infection. Infections involving the glans or prepuce are termed *balanitis* and *posthitis,* respectively. They may represent a simple bacterial infection or an inflammatory process resulting from local irritation, inspissated subpreputial secretions, or local bacterial infection. Such infections are usually treated easily with oral broad-spectrum antibiotics and better attention to local hygiene. Sometimes, recurrent balanitis may require elective circumcision if related to chronic phimosis or difficulty in retracting the foreskin. Balanitis xerotica obliterans is a chronic inflammatory condition that may cause severe induration and chronic inflammation of the glans and prepuce. This disorder is often a cause of strictures of the fossa navicularis and meatal stenosis. Treatment is complex and should be managed by a urologist; reconstructive surgery may be necessary.

Penile pain from vascular compromise may be manifested by areas of ischemia and necrosis on the glans and is most often observed in patients with advanced diabetes mellitus. Urologic consultation should be obtained for any patient in whom penile ischemia is suspected, as significant tissue loss may occur.

Urethral pain may be described as dysuria or burning on urination and may be constant or intermittent. Urethritis may reflect urethral irritation from chemical, traumatic, or infectious insults. With infectious urethritis, a urethral discharge may be present (noted by the patient as staining on undergarments) or identifiable on physical examination by digital compression of the urethra towards the meatus. Nongonococcal urethritis is most commonly due to infection with *Chlamydia* or *Mycoplasma,* may be definitively diagnosed by urethral swabs sent for appropriate microbial studies, and usually responds well to treatment with tetracycline or some of the quinolones. Gonococcal urethritis often produces a purulent discharge and significant dysuria; standard culturing and treatment regimens are applicable.

As a general note concerning sexually transmitted diseases, the specific patient complaint or physical findings on presentation may vary from a gross painless skin lesion, as with genital warts, to painful genital skin vesicles, as seen with herpes infection. Syphilis, gonorrhea, or lymphogranuloma venereum may be characterized by a classic genital chancre, dysuria, or lymphadenopathy, respectively. Diagnosis and treatment for all but the most common sexually transmitted diseases may require the expertise of a practitioner specifically knowledgeable in this area, and appropriate referral should be made if uncertainty exists.

Prostatic Pain

Pain in the perineum or prostatic region must be investigated to exclude infection, inflammatory conditions, neoplasia, and neurogenic dysfunction. Microscopic examination of expressed prostatic secretions, digital rectal examination, appropriate cultures of the urine or prostatic fluid, or from urethral swab, and other laboratory testing (such as serum prostatic specific antigen) and neurologic assessment may be necessary to assess this type of pain, which often occurs in younger men. In the absence of any identifiable abnormality or if pain is persistent after appropriate treatment, urologic referral may be indicated to further assess the patient. *Prostatodynia,* which is the term used to describe the complaint of prostatic pain without any objectively detectable abnormality, may require psychological evaluation or management but should only be used as a last resort after a thorough search for a medical or surgical explanation for the symptoms.

VOIDING SYMPTOMS

Voiding symptoms give extremely important diagnostic information in assessing urologic complaints. Coupled with a directed physical examination, a careful voiding history can help distinguish between various anatomic and functional abnormalities of the urinary tract (Table 2–1).

TABLE 2–1.
Voiding Symptoms

Obstructive Voiding Symptoms	Irritative Voiding Symptoms
Decreased force/caliber of stream	Dysuria
Hesitancy	Frequency
Incomplete emptying	Urgency
Straining to void	Nocturia
Intermittency	Urge Incontinence
Post-void dribbling	

Obstructive Symptoms

Symptoms of obstructive voiding consist of hesitancy, intermittency, straining to void, post-void dribbling, poor force and caliber of stream, and a sensation of incomplete emptying. Such symptoms are generally considered to be indicative of obstructive lesions of the bladder outlet or urethra. Common etiologies include benign prostatic hyperplasia, prostate cancer, urethral stricture disease, and bladder neck contracture. With advanced bladder outlet obstruction, continuous dribbling may occur, thereby reflecting overflow incontinence. While the aforementioned symptoms most commonly represent obstructive processes, abnormalities that cause detrusor weakness or flaccidity, such as neurogenic detrusor dysfunction, can produce similar voiding patterns. As a result, detailed history; physical findings; and, in some cases, sophisticated urodynamic studies may be necessary to distinguish between these entities.

Irritative Symptoms

Symptoms of lower urinary tract irritation include dysuria, frequency, urgency, urge incontinence, and nocturia. These symptoms represent the final common pathway of irritative foci due to a wide range of underlying processes. Common processes include urinary tract infection, foreign bodies within the bladder or urethra, bladder calculi, bladder carcinoma or carcinoma *in situ,* interstitial cystitis, and radiation cystitis. Obstructive processes can often indirectly produce irritative voiding symptoms in addition to the predictable obstructive symptoms as a reflection of progressive detrusor hypertrophy and resultant sensory and motor changes in detrusor function. Such bladder instability may be a major component of the symptom complex of bladder outlet obstruction due to benign prostatic hyperplasia (BPH) or other obstructive lesions.

Bladder instability due to neurogenic alterations may also result in irritative voiding symptoms identical to those caused by anatomic intravesical irritative foci. Voiding patterns after cerebrovascular accident, particularly when the cerebral cortex is involved, classically include significant bladder instability symptoms (often termed *uninhibited bladder* to express the loss of normal cortical control over bladder function). Diminished bladder volume from various etiologies (fibrosis, neurogenic changes) may also result in frequency, urgency, and other irritative symptoms. Pathologically increased fluid intake or output due to diabetes insipidus or syndrome of inappropriate antidiuretic hormone secretion may also result in complaints of frequency. In certain entities, such as interstitial cystitis, patients may complain of true pain with bladder filling followed by transient relief after voiding. This complaint is described as qualitatively different from typical dysuria, which is usually described as a burning sensation in the lower urinary tract during voiding.

Urinary Retention

Poor bladder emptying, determined by subjective patient report or by objective measurement of post-void residual urine volume, may be due to outflow obstruction or to poor detrusor contractility. The latter may result from detrusor decompensation after prolonged, untreated outlet obstruction or from other disease processes that result in impaired detrusor contractility. Neurologic dysfunction due to spinal cord injury, neurologic diseases, and diabetes mellitus with resultant neuropathy are common causes of inadequate bladder emptying.

Incontinence

Incontinence is classified by urologists as stress incontinence, urgency incontinence, total incontinence, and overflow incontinence. Stress incontinence, which is the loss of urine with increased intraabdominal pressure (such as straining or coughing), is most commonly noted in multiparous women due to the loss of fascial support of the bladder outlet. This loss of support allows the increases in abdominal pressure to be transmitted directly to the bladder without concomitant increase in closure pressure of the outlet. Urge incontinence occurs when patients experience the sense of urgency to void but lose urine before reaching a socially appropriate setting to void; this detrusor instability has a variety of etiologies. Total incontinence, which is the continuous loss of urine, often results from intrinsic sphincteric weakness. Overflow incontinence, as noted earlier, usually results from outlet obstruction or neurogenically related failure of bladder contractility with overflow occurring from a distended bladder. The evaluation and differential diagnosis of incontinence is discussed in detail in Chapter 5.

When a patient complains of irritative voiding, obstructive voiding, or both, a complete urologic and voiding history, urologic physical examination, neurologic history and physical examination, and functional or imaging studies may be necessary for diagnosis.

MISCELLANEOUS GENITAL COMPLAINTS
Orchialgia

Aside from the issues of differential diagnosis of scrotal pain or mass previously discussed, patients may complain of chronic or intermittent vague discomfort, aching, or sharp pains in the testicles. If a physically detectable abnormality, such as a mass, is obvious, further assessment is directed accordingly. In the absence of any physical correlate, differential diagnostic considerations include varicocele (which may be small and difficult to palpate), orchitis, atrophy, referred pain, or psychological problems. The last of these should be considered when patients complain of genital discomfort without any physical, laboratory, or imaging correlate and needs to be appropriately discussed and evaluated by a specialist if reassurance does not result in acceptable resolution of the complaint.

Small Penis

Parents may sometimes be concerned that an infant's or child's penis is smaller than they believe to be normal, or an adult patient may complain that his penis is of insufficient size. A penis smaller than two standard deviations from the norm is termed a micropenis. The normal stretched penile length for an infant is ≥1.5 cm. The mean unstretched penile length for a child aged 2 to 4 years is 3.3 ± 0.4 cm; for an adult, 12.4 cm ± 1.6 cm. Androgen replacement is the standard management for a true micropenis, and therapy is best begun before 1 year of age and preferably in infancy. The complaint of a small penis may be voiced by an adult whose penis is well within the normal range. Reassurance is generally sufficient to allay anxiety, but at times the complaint may reflect more significant sexual anxiety and psychological counseling may be indicated.

Sexual Dysfunction

Complaints related to sexual dysfunction may include loss of libido, erectile dysfunction, ejaculatory dysfunction, or genital pain or deformity during sexual activity. Loss of libido may be psychological or may be due to endocrine dysfunction. A complete medical and neurologic history and appropriate laboratory testing are necessary to properly assess loss of libido and erectile impotence. Such tests may include analysis of serum glucose concentration and levels of serum hormones, including testosterone and prolactin (to exclude testicular failure or hypothalamic-pituitary disease), assessment of nocturnal penile tumescence or duplex Doppler measurement of penile blood flow. The testing regimen can be determined on the basis of the type of treatment for which the patient is a candidate or the type in which he is interested. For example, minimal assessment might be required before offering the patient a vacuum erection device, but more extensive evaluation would be appropriate before reconstructive vascular surgery or implantation of a penile prosthesis.

Ejaculatory dysfunction includes decreasing or abnormally low ejaculate volume, absence of any antegrade ejaculate, premature ejaculation, or inability to achieve an orgasm. These issues are addressed in part in the chapters on infertility and erectile dysfunction.

HEMOSPERMIA

Blood in the ejaculate is a common and usually benign occurrence that often causes great anxiety for the patient. He should be reassured, but if the symptom recurs repeatedly he should be referred to the urologist to rule out rare but serious causes, such as chronic infection, tumor, or blood dyscrasia.

Suggested Reading

Van Arsdalen, KN: Signs and symptoms: the initial examination, in Hanno PM, Wein AJ: *Clinical Manual of Urology,* ed 2, New York, McGraw-Hill, 1994, pp 53–88.
Lowe FC, Brendler CB: Evaluation of the urologic patient, in Walsh PC and others (eds): Campbell's Urology, ed 6, Philadelphia, WB Saunders, 1992.

3

Hematuria

SIGNIFICANCE

Hematuria is indicative of potentially serious renal or urologic disease. Urinary tract cancers are the most serious conditions associated with hematuria. In 1995, an estimated 22,900 Americans will die of cancers of the urinary tract. Because urinary tract bleeding is frequently episodic, a single episode of gross hematuria should never be ignored. Urinary tract bleeding may be manifested, however, by only a few red blood cells (RBCs) detected by urinalysis. In recent studies, 39% to 90% of patients with microscopic hematuria found on screening urinalysis were not tested further. In the patients evaluated, intravenous pyelography and cystoscopy commonly were not performed. In this chapter, we discuss guidelines regarding the evaluation and differential diagnosis of hematuria and make suggestions for appropriate specialty referral.

DEFINITION

Hematuria is the abnormal presence of RBCs in the urine and is described as gross or microscopic. Gross hematuria is evident to the observer as red or rust-colored urine, and microscopic hematuria is demonstrable only under the microscope. A normal individual may excrete up to 85,000 RBCs per hour resulting in one to two RBCs per high-power field (HPF) with routine urine microscopy (40x magnification). Patients with more than three RBC/HPF on two urinalyses have significant microscopic hematuria and require further evaluation. All patients with high-grade microscopic hematuria on one urinalysis (>100 RBC/HPF) or one episode of gross hematuria require further evaluation.

URINALYSIS

Collecting the urine as well as performing and interpreting the urinalysis are of prime importance in the evaluation of the patient with hematuria. First-voided morning urine is ideal for microscopic examination because it is a concentrated specimen. Osmotic rupture of RBCs by hypotonic urine results in a positive dipstick test but a negative microscopic examination. Urinalysis is easily performed in the physician's office as described in Table 3–1.

Commercially available urine dipstick tests designed to diagnose hematuria utilize hemoglobin, from either free or intact RBCs and/or myoglobin to catalyze the conversion of an indicator dye by a peroxidase-like reaction. As few as five intact RBCs per HPF or lysed RBCs can result in a strongly positive dipstick test. A negative dipstick test correlates well with the absence of

TABLE 3–1.
Steps in Performing Routine Office Urinalysis

1. Obtain a freshly voided, midstream urine sample.
2. Describe the gross characteristics of the noncentrifuged urine regarding color and general appearance.
3. Aliquot the urine into a 10- to 15-ml tube and centrifuge for 3-5 minutes at 2000-3000 rpm.
4. Perform a dipstick test on the remaining urine sample.
5. Decant the supernatant and resuspend the sediment.
6. Pipette or pour a drop on a microscope slide and place a cover slip.
7. Examine the specimen under 10x (low power) and 40x (high power).
8. Record the number of RBCs and WBCs/HPF and note the presence of casts, crystals, and bacteria.

significant microscopic hematuria on urinalysis. In a double-blind study of 1346 asymptomatic patients, 9% of patients with more than two RBC/HPF had a negative dipstick test and 84% of patients with more than three RBC/HPF had a positive dipstick test.

For screening purposes, the dipstick test rules out significant hematuria with 99% accuracy, but the presence of a positive dipstick reading requires microscopic examination of the urine. A strongly positive dipstick test with no RBCs identified by microscopy may result from sampling errors; lysis of RBCs by hypotonic urine; and, rarely, hemoglobinuria or myoglobinuria. In this situation, urinalysis should be repeated with a sample of first-voided morning urine. Hemoglobinuria and myoglobinuria are diagnoses of exclusion and do not require further urologic evaluation.

ASSOCIATED MICROSCOPIC FINDINGS
Red Blood Cell Casts

Microscopy of urinary sediment allows for identification of RBC casts that are suggestive of glomerular bleeding. The RBC casts result from precipitation of Tamm-Horsfall mucoprotein within the renal tubule and trapping of clusters of RBCs (Fig. 3–1A). While RBC casts strongly support the diagnosis of glomerular bleeding, these casts are often not detected on urinalysis because they are fragile. The use of low-speed centrifugation (1000 rpm for 2 minutes) or even gravity sedimentation for 30 minutes will enhance the detection rate. When

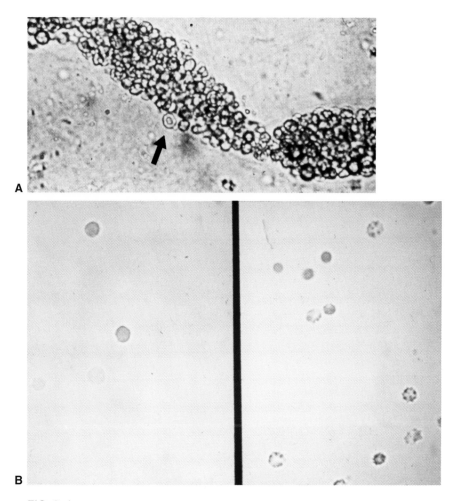

FIG. 3–1.

A, Red blood cell cast in a patient with glomerular hematuria. **B,** Red blood cells of uniform morphology consistent with an epithelial origin *(left panel).* Normal and crenated red blood cells, which may represent upper urinary tract bleeding in a freshly voided urine sample *(right panel).*

RBC casts are present with significant proteinuria, a diagnosis of glomerular hematuria is more likely. RBC casts are seen with acute interstitial nephritis, glomerulonephritis, diabetic nephropathy, renal vein thrombosis, and even exercise. Patients with RBC casts should be referred to a nephrologist for further evaluation, which may include renal biopsy, and for appropriate management.

Red Blood Cell Morphology

RBC morphology can help distinguish glomerular (renal) from nonglomerular (epithelial) bleeding. Urinary RBCs of varied sizes, shapes, and hemoglobin distribution are considered dysmorphic and are indicative of glomerular or possibly tubulointerstitial disease, while those of uniform morphology with an even hemoglobin distribution are considered isomorphic and are indicative of epithelial origin (Fig. 3–1*B*). In questionable cases, inspection of urine sediment by phase-contrast microscopy or the determination of urinary RBC size distribution curves using a Coulter counter may determine RBC morphology with greater accuracy than light microscopy alone.

Proteinuria

Healthy adults excrete approximately 80 to 150 milligrams of protein daily. A patient with hematuria associated with greater than 2+ proteinuria detected by a dipstick test should complete a 24-hour urine collection for quantitative protein excretion and creatinine clearance determination. If the total protein is greater than 150 milligrams, further evaluation to rule out glomerular or tubulointerstitial disease should be considered.

Pyuria

Significant pyuria is more than three white blood cells (WBC)/HPF and is indicative of urinary tract inflammation, infection, or both. Pyuria is detectable by a leukocyte esterase dipstick test and should be confirmed by light microscopy. When hematuria is associated with pyuria, an infectious etiology should be strongly considered. Therefore, a urine culture and sensitivity test should be obtained and antimicrobial treatment initiated according to the culture results. If the hematuria clears along with the pyuria after antimicrobial treatment, acute bacterial cystitis should be considered the most likely source of bleeding, and the patient is followed appropriately.

Patients with recurrent culture-proven infection of the urinary tract should be referred to a urologist for further evaluation, which usually includes an upper urinary tract study (renal ultrasonography and plane radiograph of the abdomen (KUB) or intravenous urogram) and cystoscopy. Sterile pyuria is classically associated with genitourinary tuberculosis but may also occur in the setting of urinary tract neoplasia or calculi. An intravenous urogram usually identifies the cause, and cystoscopy should be performed to examine the urethra and bladder.

HISTORY AND PHYSICAL EXAMINATION

A thorough history and physical examination will provide valuable information regarding the most likely source of urinary tract bleeding. A differential diagnosis focused on the upper or lower urinary tract enables the physician to conduct a cost-effective and efficient evaluation. Hematuria in children is alarming but is very often benign and self-limited. The likelihood that hematuria signifies serious urologic disease increases sharply after 50 years of age. Patient gender affects the likelihood of underlying malignancy, as men are affected by urinary tract cancers more than twice as often as women. Table 3–2 illustrates the most common causes of hematuria by age and sex.

Characterization of Hematuria

The history should clearly establish whether hematuria is gross or microscopic. In general, the degree of hematuria increases with the likelihood of serious pathology. Gross hematuria is further characterized with regard to the portion of the urinary stream involved. If hematuria is noted at the beginning of urination, the urethra or prostate is the most likely source. If hematuria is observed at the end of voiding, the trigone or bladder neck is the most likely source. Total gross hematuria observed throughout voiding indicates that the source of bleeding is the bladder, ureter, or kidney. If there is evidence of urinary clot retention, a large-caliber Foley catheter should be used to drain the patient's bladder. All clots should be removed from the bladder through irrigation, and a urologist should be consulted for immediate evaluation and treatment. An intravenous urogram is obtained, and cystoscopy is required to observe the source of bleeding and to determine appropriate therapy. In female patients, cyclic hematuria occurring with menses suggests endometriosis of the urinary tract.

Pseudohematuria should be ruled out in patients who report signs consistent with gross hematuria. Many urinary pigments impart a red color to the urine, mimicking gross hematuria. Excessive consumption of beets or berries containing anthocyanins, food coloring (rhodamine B), laxatives (phenolphthalein), urinary tract analgesics (phenazopyridine), and rifampin may give the urine a red appearance despite a negative urine dipstick test. Once pseudohematuria is clearly established by normal urinalysis results, no further evaluation is warranted and the patient can be reassured.

In men, it is important that the history clarifies the difference between gross hematuria and hematospermia, or blood in the semen. Hemospermia in young adult males is a sign of seminal vesicle inflammation, and a single episode is generally little cause for concern. Acute prostatitis or seminal vesiculitis is the most common cause in men younger than 40 years of age and is effectively

TABLE 3–2.
Common Causes of Hematuria by Age and Sex

0–20 Years
- Poststreptococcal glomerulonephritis
- Acute urinary tract infection
- Orthostatic hematuria related to heavy exercise
- Congenital renal anomalies (ureteropelvic junction obstruction, multicystic dysplastic kidney)
- Malignant neoplasm (Wilm's tumor, rhabdomyosarcoma, leiomyosarcoma, renal cell carcinoma, transitional cell carcinoma)

20–40 years
- Acute urinary tract infection
- Urolithiasis
- Benign recurrent hematuria
- Bladder tumor

40–60 years (Males)
- Bladder tumor
- Urolithiasis
- Acute urinary tract infection
- Renal tumors

40–60 years (Females)
- Acute urinary tract infection
- Urolithiasis
- Bladder tumor
- Renal tumors

60 years/over (Males)
- Benign prostatic hyperplasia
- Bladder tumor
- Acute urinary tract infection

60 years (Females)
- Bladder tumor
- Acute urinary tract infection

treated with tetracycline or erythromycin. In older patients, hemospermia may be indicative of prostate cancer with seminal vesicle involvement. A prostate specific antigen (PSA) test should be obtained, and a careful digital rectal examination (DRE) of the prostate should be performed. Patients with an elevated PSA or abnormal DRE should be referred to a urologist for consideration of a prostate biopsy. Transrectal ultrasonography is not used routinely for early detection of prostate cancer but is very useful in conjunction with prostate biopsy and for staging of prostate cancer.

Exercise-induced hematuria should be considered in adolescents and young adults. Intrarenal hypoxia and efferent arteriolar constriction during exercise may result in increased excretion of RBCs. Gross hematuria has been reported in long-distance runners with mirror-image contusions of the trigone and dome of the bladder presumably due to multiple impacts of the fixed trigone on the mobile bladder dome. This is a diagnosis of exclusion and does not require further evaluation.

Associated Symptoms

Irritative voiding symptoms, such as painful urination and urgency and frequency of urination, are indicative of an inflammatory condition of the bladder, prostate, or urethra. A urine culture should be obtained and infection treated with appropriate antibiotics. Hematuria with irritative voiding symptoms is also a frequent finding in patients with bladder cancer. Urine cytology obtained via catheter lavage of the bladder with normal saline is very sensitive for the detection of carcinoma *in situ* and high-grade bladder cancer. Such obstructive voiding symptoms as decreased force of the urinary stream, hesitancy, and incomplete emptying of the bladder are additional clues that suggest lower urinary tract pathology. Flank pain indicates that the kidney or ureter is the most likely source of urinary tract bleeding. Abdominal pain or an ileus may result from inflammation of the kidney or ureter due to infection, neoplasia, or trauma. Fever may be associated with neoplasia or infection and indicates that the kidney or ureter is the most likely site of pathology.

Medical and Surgical History

The clinician should inquire about a history of urolithiasis, urinary tract malignancy, or urologic surgery. Other conditions, such as primary renal disease, systemic lupus erythematosus, Henoch-Schönlein purpura, Goodpasture's syndrome, and membranoproliferative glomerulonephritis, may be associated with hematuria. The clinician should inquire about recent illnesses. For instance, grossly bloody urine within a day or two of an upper respiratory illness suggests IgA nephropathy (or Berger's disease). A lag time of two to three weeks between pharyngitis and onset of gross hematuria suggests post-streptococcal glomerulonephritis. In such cases, an antistreptolysin O (ASO) titer is helpful in confirming the diagnosis.

Medications

Current and past use of medication may provide clues to the etiology of hematuria. Hematuria associated with use of anticoagulants or nonsteroidal anti-inflammatory agents is associated with significant urinary tract disease in up to 50% of patients and always requires further evaluation (i.e., an IVP and cystoscopy) to elicit the cause. The cytotoxic chemotherapy agents cyclophosphamide and ifosfamide cause hemorrhagic cystitis due to the metabolite acrolein that is excreted by the kidneys, and these agents are also associated with an increased risk of bladder cancer. Phenacetin is an aniline derivative that is known to cause urothelial carcinoma. Large doses of vitamin C may cause hyperoxaluria, which increases the risk of calcium oxalate stone formation in the urinary tract.

Social History

The clinician should be aware of important risk factors for urinary tract malignancy that can be elicited with a careful social and occupational history. Environmental carcinogen exposure induces up to 50% of urothelial carcinoma. Cigarette smoking is by far the most common urothelial carcinogen and is estimated to account for as much as 47% of cases of bladder cancer in men and 37% in women. Cigarette smoking is also associated with renal cell carcinoma, causing 30% of the cases documented in men and 24% in women. Other occupational risk factors for urinary tract malignancy include exposure to aromatic amines, such as aniline dyes, benzidine, and naphthylamine. The latency period from exposure to clinically detectable cancer can be as long as 25 years.

Family History

Many inheritable conditions specifically affect the urinary tract and may cause hematuria. Familial nephritis (Alport's syndrome) and polycystic kidney disease may cause renal hematuria. Hematuria may be the presenting sign in patients with familial forms of renal cell carcinoma, including von Hippel Lindau disease. Cystinuria and hereditary oxaluria cause urinary tract calculi, which are a frequent cause of hematuria. Patients with sickle cell disease or those who carry the trait are prone to renal injury when sickle cells become trapped in small vessels and cause thrombosis and infarction. Papillary necrosis is a common complication of sickle cell nephropathy that causes hematuria and possible obstruction of the urinary tract by a sloughed papilla. Essential hematuria is a diagnosis of exclusion and may be associated with a familial predisposition.

Trauma

Traumatic injury to the urinary tract is classified as penetrating or blunt. Hematuria is a constant finding with penetrating injuries of the urinary tract with the exception of renal hilar injuries. The degree of hematuria does not necessarily correlate with the severity of the injury. An intravenous urogram is used to assess function of both kidneys and, in hemodynamically stable patients, nephrotomography or computed tomography adequately stages a renal injury.

Gross hematuria associated with blunt trauma to the abdomen is best evaluated with computed tomography. A stress cystogram is the best method for evaluating the bladder for injury and should be performed in patients with injuries to the pelvis or lower abdomen. Hemodynamically stable adult patients with microscopic hematuria and no hypotension prior to arrival in the emergency room can be observed without radiographic evaluation. The urologist is an integral part of the surgical team in the evaluation of traumatically injured patients and should be consulted immediately when urinary tract injury is suspected to establish an appropriate management plan. Additional studies, including renal arteriography, may be required. Surgical exploration and repair of an injured kidney is reserved for patients with persistent bleeding and/or devascularization of a significant portion of the kidney.

Physical Examination

A careful assessment of the patient's vital signs provides clues to the etiology of hematuria. Fever and tachycardia suggest infection, such as pyelonephritis, or neoplasia, such as renal cell carcinoma. Hypertension is associated with glomerulonephritis and, in children, frequently accompanies pyelonephritis or hydronephrosis. A thorough physical examination is important to detect diseases that may secondarily affect the urinary tract. Examples include Alport's syndrome (nephritis and hearing loss), von Hippel Lindau disease (manifestations include cerebellar and spinal cord hemangioblastomas, retinal hemangioma, pheochromocytoma, and renal cell carcinoma), and tuberous sclerosis (manifestations include mental retardation, adenoma sebaceum, and renal angiomyolipoma).

The physical examination is directed to the urinary tract, with careful examination and inspection of the abdomen, external genitalia, pelvis (by means of bimanual examination), and rectum. The extremities should be examined to rule out edema and skin or joint abnormalities, which can indicate various renal diseases. When trauma is suspected, the back and flank are inspected for ecchymosis, and the pelvic bones are examined for possible fracture. Blood at the urethral meatus implies a urethral injury until proven otherwise.

DIFFERENTIAL DIAGNOSIS

A carefully performed history, physical examination, and urinalysis provide a wealth of information that helps the physician localize the bleeding to the upper or lower urinary tract and formulate an appropriate differential diagnosis. Table 3–3 provides a detailed differential diagnosis of the diseases of the renal parenchyma, urinary tract collecting system, and lower urinary tract to be considered in patients with hematuria. The following is a discussion of some of the more common entities and a practical method of evaluation.

Glomerular Hematuria

The diagnosis of glomerular hematuria is suggested by the presence of dysmorphic RBCs and RBC casts as well as significant proteinuria. Hypertension may also provide another clue. Initial studies should include serum chemistries and measurement of blood urea nitrogen and creatinine levels as well as a 24-hour urine collection for quantitative protein excretion and creatinine clearance determination. The most common glomerular disorders found in a review of 151 patients are listed in Table 3–4 on page 40. Consultation with a nephrologist is important when glomerular hematuria is suspected to select appropriate therapy and determine whether renal biopsy is necessary.

Berger's disease is suggested by gross hematuria following an upper respiratory tract infection or exercise and is most common in children and young adult males. Kidney function usually remains normal but microscopic hematuria may persist. Advanced age at onset, heavy proteinuria, hypertension, and diminished renal function are associated with a poor prognosis. Renal insufficiency is observed in 25% of patients with Berger's disease. Diagnosis is validated by kidney biopsy and immunofluorescent studies.

Mesangioproliferative glomerulonephritis is more common in children than in adults. Males are more commonly affected by familial nephritis or Alport's syndrome. This disease is associated with hearing loss, but the nephrotic syndrome is rare. In the pediatric population, poststreptococcal glomerulonephritis is a common cause of glomerular hematuria. Patients with congenital anomalies (including ureteropelvic junction obstruction and anomalies of size, shape, or location) may present with hematuria as the initial manifestation, particularly in association with trauma.

TABLE 3–3.
Hematuria Differential Diagnosis*

I. RENAL PARENCHYMAL DISEASES
  A. Glomerular Disease
    1. Primary Renal Disease
      a. Idiopathic recurrent hematuria
      b. Berger's disease
      c. Resolving postinfectious glomerulonephritis
      d. Membranoproliferative glomerulonephritis
      e. Focal glomerulosclerosis
      f. Crescentic glomerulonephritis
      g. Minimal change disease
      h. Membranous nephropathy
      i. Mesangial proliferative glomerulonephritis (including IgM nephropathy)
      j. Focal and segmental proliferative glomerulonephritis
    2. Multisystem or Hereditary Disease
      a. Systemic lupus erythematosus
      b. Vasculitis (including Wegener's granulomatosis)
      c. Schönlein-Henoch purpura
      d. Goodpasture's syndrome
      e. Infective endocarditis and sepsis
      f. Alport's syndrome
      g. Fabry's disease
      h. Nail-patella syndrome
      i. Thrombotic microangiopathies (hemolytic uremia syndrome, thrombotic thrombocytopenic purpura)
      j. Amyloidosis (rare)
    3. Malignant hypertension
    4. Jogger's or Marathon Runner's Hematuria (?)
  B. Non-Glomerular
    1. Acute hypersensitivity interstitial nephros

  2. Polycystic kidney disease
  3. Medullary sponge kidney
  4. Papillary necrosis (e.g., analgesic abuse, sickle cell trait, diabetes mellitus, alcoholism
  5. Trauma
  6. Tumors (renal cell carcinoma, Wilm's tumor)
  7. Leukemic infiltrates
  8. Vascular anomalies
  9. Severe hydronephrosis
  10. Renal infarction (emboli or thrombosis)
  11. Renal vein thrombosis
  12. Hypercalciuria
  13. Loin pain-hematuria syndrome

II. EXTRA-RENAL PARENCHYMAL
  A. Ureter
    1. Calculi (uric acid, cystine, xanthine, Ca oxalate, Ca phosphate, triple phosphate dihydroxyadenine)
    2. Tumors
    3. Peri-urethritis (appendicitis, retroperitoneal abscess, ileocolitis)
    4. Retroperitoneal fibrosis
    5. Ureterocele
    6. Varices
    7. Ureteritis (tuberculosis, etc.)
    8. Endometriosis
  B. Bladder
    1. Cystitis (bacterial, viral, parasitic, fungal)
    2. Chronic interstitial cystitis (Hunner's ulcers)
    3. Radiation cystitis
    4. Nitrogen mustard or cyclophosphamide cystitis
    5. Hypersensitivity (allergic) cystitis

(continued)

TABLE 3–3. *(Continued)*
Hematuria Differential Diagnosis*

6. Carcinoma of the bladder
7. Calculi
8. Trauma
9. Jogger's or Marathon's
    Runner's hematuria (?)
10. Vascular anomalies
11. Foreign bodies
12. Endometriosis
C. Prostate
    1. Benign prostatic hypertrophy
    2. Carcinoma of the prostate
    3. Chronic or acute prostatitis
D. Urethra
    1. Meatal ulcers
    2. Prolapse
    3. Carbuncle
    4. Acute or chronic urethritis
       (bacterial, viral)
    5. Carcinoma
    6. Vascular anomalies
    7. Trauma
    8. Foreign bodies
    9. Condyloma acuminata

III. RELATED TO A SYSTEMIC
     COAGULATION DISTURBANCE
     (with or without additional disease in
     previous list)
     A. Platelet Defect
        1. Idiopathic or drug induced
           thrombocytopenic purpura
        2. Thromboasthenia
        3. Bone marrow infiltration with
           thrombocytopenia
     B. Coagulation Protein Deficiency
        1. Hemophilia A or B
        2. Heparin therapy
        3. Oral anticoagulants
        4. Other congenital and acquired
           disturbances of coagulation
     C. Other
        1. Scurvy
        2. Hereditary telangiectasis
IV. IDIOPATHIC
    A. "Benign Recurrent Hematuria"
       1. Familial
       2. Sporadic

From Glassock RJ: The evaluation of hematuria and proteinuria, AUA Update, vol III(30), 1984. Adapted with permission.

Nonglomerular Renal Hematuria

In adult patients, the physician must identify or rule out malignancy as the cause of hematuria. The most common solid renal neoplasm is renal cell carcinoma. Other renal parenchymal tumors include sarcomas, oncocytoma, and benign angiomyolipomas. Diagnosis is established by intravenous urography and computed tomography. Transitional cell carcinomas may arise anywhere in the urinary tract and appear as a filling defect on intravenous urography. Referral to a urologist is appropriate in order to establish the diagnosis by positive urinary cytology and endoscopic visualization and/or biopsy.

Urinary tract calculi are invariably associated with hematuria. Flank pain suggests obstruction and hydronephrosis and the pain frequently radiates to the lower abdomen. Irritative voiding symptoms suggest a distal ureteral stone. Patients with hydronephrosis and infection should be referred immediately to a

TABLE 3–4.

Glomerular Disorders in 151 Patients with Glomerular Hematuria*

Disorder	Percentage of Patients	Percentage of Patients with Hematuria Alone†
IgA nephropathy (Berger's disease)	30	23
Mesangioproliferative GN	14	31
Focal segmental proliferative GN	13	27
Familial nephritis (Alport's syndrome)	11	23
Membranous GN	7	0
Mesangiocapillary GN	6	0
Focal segmental sclerosis	4	0
Unclassifiable	4	0
Systemic lupus erythematosus	3	0
Postinfectious GN	2	100
Subacute bacterial endocarditis	2	100
Others	4	0
Total	100	21

*From Fassett RG and others: Detection of glomerular bleeding by phase-contrast microscopy. Lancet 1:1432, 1982. Adapted with permission.
†Patients with glomerular hematuria not accompanied by red blood cell casts or proteinuria.
GN = glomerulonephritis.

urologist to undergo ureteral stent placement or percutaneous nephrostomy to relieve the obstruction.

Patients with end-stage renal disease who develop acquired cystic disease of the kidneys (ACDK) are particularly at risk for renal cell carcinoma. Most patients with ACDK are treated with hemodialysis; however, some are treated with peritoneal dialysis and others are never dialyzed. The estimated incidence of ACDK from cumulative series is 45% for patients with end-stage renal disease, and the relative risk of renal cell carcinoma in patients with ACDK is reported to be as high as 41 times that of the general population. Screening for ACDK should be performed with ultrasonography at the initiation of dialysis and continued every two years. Computed tomography should be done for any patient with hematuria or a solid lesion suspected on ultrasonography.

Renal artery embolism and thrombosis may occur following blunt trauma to the abdomen, manipulation of the aorta during angiography or surgery, or spontaneously. Microscopic or gross hematuria and mild proteinuria are observed in only about one half of patients. All or a part of the kidney may not be visualized by intravenous urography.

Renal arteriovenous fistulas may be congenital or acquired and may be associated with hematuria, cardiac failure due to increased cardiac output, and hypertension. A flank or abdominal bruit may be present, and the intravenous urogram is frequently normal. The diagnosis is suggested by recurrent unilateral gross hematuria and is confirmed by renal angiography. Treatment is generally accomplished by angiographic embolization of the branch renal artery.

Renal vein thrombosis in infants may arise bilaterally as a result of severe dehydration due to diarrhea or vomiting. In adult patients, the disorder is often unilateral and associated with the nephrotic syndrome. The kidney frequently is enlarged, and hematuria due to focal renal infarction is common. Computed tomography and magnetic resonance imaging may demonstrate an enlarged kidney and thrombosis of the renal vein. In children, acute thrombosis is associated with severe flank pain, hypertension, and shock and is frequently fatal.

Lower Urinary Tract Hematuria

Benign prostatic hyperplasia is the most common cause of hematuria in men older than 50 years of age. This is a diagnosis of exclusion, however, as absence of malignancy must be proven first. Prostate cancer is frequently asymptomatic, but advanced cases may be associated with hematuria or hemospermia. Men younger than 70 years of age with an elevated PSA or abnormal digital rectal examination should be referred to a urologist for consideration of prostate biopsy. Bladder cancer is the fifth most common solid tumor malignancy in adults and affects men three times as often as women. A filling defect in the bladder may be observed on intravenous urography, and the diagnosis is confirmed by the urologist with cystoscopy and urine cytology.

HEMATURIA EVALUATION

Initial studies should include a urine culture to rule out infection as the cause for hematuria as well as to determine blood urea nitrogen and serum creatinine. Adult patients with significant hematuria who have creatinine values lower than 1.8 mg/dl and no contrast allergy should undergo an intravenous urogram. This study should include nephrotomograms in order to completely visualize the renal parenchyma.

Adult patients with unexplained gross or microscopic hematuria should undergo cystoscopic examination. Cystourethroscopy is the only reliable means of evaluating the bladder and the urethra. This is a short procedure performed by a urologist in the office setting using a small-caliber rigid or flexible fiber-optic instrument, which causes minimal discomfort to the patient. With unexplained hematuria, a barbotage bladder washing obtained at the time of cystoscopy is recommended to rule out carcinoma *in situ* of the bladder. Voided urine cytology is not as sensitive as bladder washings obtained by the barbotage technique—the latter method has a sensitivity of 67% and specificity of 96% for the detection of urothelial cancer. Sterility of the urine should be confirmed by urine culture prior to cystoscopy.

Contrast-induced renal failure occurs in 0.8% of patients without preexisting renal disease and in up to 50% of patients with renal impairment due to diabetes mellitus or multiple myeloma. Patients with renal insufficiency or those who are allergic to iodinated contrast material should undergo renal ultrasonography and a KUB instead of an intravenous urogram as the initial screening radiographic study. These studies provide excellent visualization of the renal parenchyma and reliably identify radiopaque calculi within the urinary tract. Visualization of the collecting system of the urinary tract is provided by retrograde ureteropyelography done at the time of cystoscopy. These studies are performed by the urologist in an outpatient surgical setting.

If a renal mass is detected by intravenous urography, renal ultrasonography will determine whether it is cystic or solid. If the mass is a complex cyst or a solid mass, computed tomography with and without intravenous contrast should be performed. The patient should then be referred to a urologist for further evaluation and possible surgical management. An asymptomatic patient with a simple benign cyst can be followed by the primary-care physician.

When a thorough evaluation fails to demonstrate an etiology for hematuria, a renal arteriogram can be performed to rule out a renal arteriovenous malformation, especially when unilateral gross hematuria is noted on cystoscopy. Furthermore, ureteroscopy can be used to further evaluate a radiographically apparent ureteral or renal pelvis lesion or to perform a biopsy.

Although urologic malignancy is rare in children, a child who presents with hematuria should be evaluated. Pediatric patients with unexplained hematuria should undergo renal ultrasonography to rule out congenital or neoplastic renal diseases. If the renal sonogram is normal and hematuria persists, consideration should be given to cystoscopy to rule out pathology of the lower urinary tract.

CONCLUSION

Hematuria is an alarming finding for both the clinician and the patient. A few RBCs on microscopic urinalysis may be the only sign of serious disease of the urinary tract. A systematic approach guided by a thorough history and physical examination, followed by a carefully performed urinalysis, often gives significant clues to the most likely source of the bleeding. The age and sex of the patient, as well as associated symptoms, greatly assist the physician in formulating a differential diagnosis and in choosing the appropriate tests to discern the source of the bleeding. This logical approach should ensure an adequate and cost-effective evaluation of hematuria and provide a guide to appropriate nephrologic or urologic referrals.

Suggested Reading

Abarbanel J and others: Sports hematuria, *J Urol* 143:887–890, 1990.

Birch DF and others: Urinary erythrocyte morphology in the diagnosis of glomerular hematuria, *Clin Nephrol* 20:78–85, 1983.

Fallon B, Williams RD: Renal cancer associated with acquired cystic disease of the kidney and chronic renal failure, *Semin Urol* 7(4):228–236, 1989.

Glassock JR: The evaluation of hematuria and proteinuria, *AUA—Update Series,* vol III(30), 1984.

Lerner SP, Eastham J: Cancers of the urinary tract, in Suki W, Massry S (eds): *Therapy of Renal Diseases and Related Disorders, ed 3.* Boston, Kluwer Academic Publishers, 1995.

Mariani JA: The evaluation of adult hematuria, *AUA—Update Series* VIII(23), 1989.

Mee SL and others: Radiographic assessment of renal trauma: A 10 year prospective study of patient selection, *J Urol* 141:1095, 1989.

Schuster AG, Lewis AG: Clinical significance of hematuria in patients on anticoagulant therapy, *J Urol* 137:923, 1987.

Shichiri M and others: Red cell volume distribution curves in diagnosis of glomerular and non glomerular hematuria, *Lancet* 1:908–911, 1988.

Sutton J: Evaluation of hematuria in adults, *JAMA* 263(18): 2475, 1990.

Williams AM, Noe HN: Childhood hematuria: deciding when it's serious, *Contemp Urol* January:29–37, 1993.

Wingo PA, Tong T, Bolden S: Cancer statistics, 1995, *Ca Cancer J Clin* 45:8–30, 1995.

4

Recurrent Urinary Tract Infection

Recurrent urinary tract infection (UTI) is a significant source of morbidity in our country today. The incidence, pathogenesis, and treatment of recurring UTI vary with the age and gender of the patients being studied. The management of UTI in the ambulatory, outpatient setting can best be addressed by separate discussions of treatment of women, men, and children, with particular emphasis placed on that group most at risk: premenopausal females.

RECURRENT URINARY TRACT INFECTION IN WOMEN
Premenopausal Women

At least one-third of the women in the United States experience uncomplicated acute UTI, with most of these individuals having the initial bout after puberty. We now recognize that the bacteria infecting the urinary tracts of such women usually come from fecal flora. Sexual activity is a primary risk factor for symptomatic UTI, with the relative risk depending on the actual sexual practice as well as frequency and timing. The 48-hour period after vaginal intercourse is the window of highest risk. Use of oral contraceptives, urination before sex, frequency of washing, direction of wiping after a bowel movement, and use of tampons do not appear to affect the risk for UTI, after adjustment for other risk factors. Urination after sex, however, does seem to reduce risk. Diaphragm use increases the risk for bacteriuria but not for symptomatic UTI. Increasing age and prior history of UTI are associated with slightly increased risk.

Approximately 20% of women who have had one episode of UTI experience a recurrence. Susceptibility to recurrent UTI is mainly characterized by abnormally high numbers of fecal bacteria on the vaginal and urethral mucosa. The high numbers are apparently related to increased bacterial attachment to squamous epithelial cell receptors; the occurrence is influenced by genetic factors that persist despite fluctuation in patient susceptibility.

When a UTI recurs, it is important to first determine that unresolved, or incompletely treated, bacteriuria is not the underlying problem. Bacterial resistance is the most common reason for drug failure.

If bacteriuria has resolved and the UTI recurs, either persistence or reinfection is responsible. Persistence is recurrence of the UTI from a site within the urinary tract. In women, persistence can result from stones, fistulae, diverticulae, or other relatively rare urologic abnormalities. Reinfection, on the other hand, arises from a site outside the urinary tract. Reinfection is far more common than persistence as a cause of recurring UTI in women. This should not be surprising, considering the length of the female urethra and the proximity of the urethral meatus to the colonized vaginal mucosa.

Diagnosis and Work-Up

It has been demonstrated that between 20% and 40% of women with symptomatic UTI present with bacterial counts of less than 10^5/ml of urine. In dysuric patients, a more appropriate threshold value for defining significant bacteriuria is 10^2 colonies/ml of a known pathogen in a catheterized urine specimen. With recurring UTI, this pathogen is very likely to be *Escherichia coli.* Screening urinalysis nearly always reveals significant pyuria, thus allowing physicians to begin treatment presumptively. Urinalysis also helps differentiate recurrent UTI from other noninflammatory causes of dysuric symptoms in females.

Indications for urologic imaging and cystoscopy in premenopausal women are not clearly defined and are determined primarily by the clinical impression of the physician. The typical recurrence due to reinfection is related causally to intercourse and involves *E. coli.* Atypical features include infection with urea-splitting bacteria, obstructive voiding complaints, and such symptoms of upper tract involvement as flank pain. Suspicion of persistence, rather than reinfection, should arise if the UTI recurs within two weeks after treatment. Any such findings should alert the practitioner to the possibility of an anatomic or structural cause of the recurrence and aid in selecting such patients with recurring UTI who need urologic referral.

Treatment

As noted, some women are biologically predisposed to recurrent UTI resulting from vaginal and periurethral colonization with fecal flora. Understanding of this process has led to phase I clinical trials using heat-killed, vaginally applied strains of coliform bacteria as immunization against recurring UTI. This treatment has been well tolerated and has proved capable of increasing vaginal and urinary antibodies; however, efficacy has yet to be demonstrated.

Recognition of behavioral risk factors has allowed us to advise women that discontinuing diaphragm use and voiding after sexual intercourse can diminish recurrences. These nonpharmacologic means, however, are often insufficient in helping women whose predisposition to infection persists despite changes in life-style. It should be noted that abstaining from intercourse does prevent development of new UTI in these women, but such measures are impractical for most patients.

Antibiotic prophylaxis is the most practical preventive measure for most women. Because as many as 85% of women with recurrent UTI have onset of symptoms within 24 hours of intercourse, postcoital use of antibiotics should be tried before long daily courses are used. Randomized, double-blind, controlled trials using a variety of drugs have demonstrated the efficacy of such an approach.

Trimethoprim-sulfamethoxazole, nitrofurantoin, quinolones, cephalosporins, and sulfisoxazole have all been used for postcoital prophylaxis. The first three agents have been particularly successful; thus, the decision to treat daily should be made only if the postcoital approach has failed.

Despite reported successes, the choice of an antibiotic is not straightforward. Earlier trials between trimethoprim-sulfamethoxazole and nitrofurantoin demonstrated similar success rates, despite concerns regarding the ability of trimethoprim-sulfamethoxazole to select out resistant strains of bowel and vaginal flora. Nitrofurantoin, although it does not alter bowel flora, has been shown to cause irreversible pulmonary fibrosis with long-term daily use in some patients and is no longer recommended by some physicians. The quinolones seem to have slightly greater efficacy, although at an increased cost. These agents not only sterilize urine but also clear most of the introital and urethral flora. As yet, there have been no reports that women who consistently take a single dose of quinolone after intercourse develop resistant organisms.

In patients refractory to postcoital prophylaxis and electing to proceed with daily medication, an initial trial of 6 to 12 months of treatment is recommended. Some patients demonstrate sustained clinical improvement, and infection does not recur.

Postmenopausal Women

Circulating estrogens encourage colonization of the vagina by lactobacilli. These bacteria produce lactic acid from glycogen and maintain a low vaginal pH that inhibits the growth of many bacterial pathogens. In the absence of intercourse, this mechanism is effective in keeping urine sterile despite the bladder's proximity to the perineum.

An estimated 10% to 15% of women older than 60 years of age have frequent UTI. Postmenopausal changes in vaginal flora due to lack of circulating estrogens are believed to play a primary role in this high incidence. Postmenopausal vaginal pH increases with the disappearance of lactobacilli, and the vagina is colonized with Enterobacteriaceae, especially *E. coli.*

Treatment in Postmenopausal Women

Treatment of recurrent UTI in this age group has focused on estrogen-replacement therapy. Several studies using oral estriol suggest efficacy in prevention of recurrent UTI. One large, case-controlled study, however, found that oral estrogen use was associated with a twofold increase in the risk of a first episode of UTI. Other concerns about effects of systemic estrogens in this age group also remain unresolved. For these reasons, a randomized, double-blind, controlled trial was recently undertaken using topically applied estriol cream. This regimen effectively lowered vaginal pH, increased colonization with lactobacilli, and lowered colonization rates of Enterobacteriaceae without producing systemic estrogen effects. Most important, the incidence of UTI was significantly reduced over that found with placebo.

Vaginally applied estrogens seem to be an appropriate initial treatment for many postmenopausal women, although daily, low-dose, antibiotic prophylaxis still plays a role in many patients. Studies conducted for periods of several years have demonstrated continued long-term efficacy of many drugs with little evidence of increasing rates of toxicity or bacterial resistance.

Pregnant Women

The prevalence of recurrent UTI among pregnant women is similar to that among sexually active, nonpregnant, premenopausal women. UTI during pregnancy, however, progresses to acute pyelonephritis in about one-third of cases. This high rate of progression probably is related to upper tract dilation and the resultant stasis often seen in the later stages of pregnancy.

The obvious morbidity of a febrile upper UTI during pregnancy has led to increased efforts to prevent lower tract infections in pregnant women. The data showing similar rates of UTI in pregnant and nonpregnant women in addition to the finding that as many as 43% of women who develop UTI during pregnancy have a history of UTI before pregnancy seem to point to a common mechanism of infection for all premenopausal females, regardless of pregnancy status.

Treatment in Pregnant Women

Many antibacterial treatment regimens have been suggested for recurrent UTI during pregnancy. Certainly, asymptomatic bacteriuria constitutes an indication for treatment in this high-risk group. Many believe that prophylaxis should begin after treatment of the first UTI of pregnancy, especially if the patient has a history of UTI. The optimal course of treatment, including choice of drug and length of therapy, is still controversial. However, most obstetricians recommend nitrofurantoin or a penicillin to control UTI during pregnancy

As in other premenopausal females who experience UTI after intercourse, postcoital antibacterial prophylaxis has been studied in pregnant women as first-line therapy to prevent recurrence. This seems to be at least as effective as daily, single-dose therapy. In a recent study of 39 women who had a total of 130 UTIs during a prepregnancy observation period, one person was reported to have experienced UTI during pregnancy after treatment was begun. A single, low dose of either cephalexin or nitrofurantoin was used. A benefit of postcoital therapy was the minimal amount of drug required when compared with daily dosing. It is likely that either trimethoprim-sulfamethoxazole or nitrofurantoin would be effective in this role, but it should be noted that only cephalosporins and penicillins are known to be safe at all stages of pregnancy.

RECURRENT URINARY TRACT INFECTION IN MEN

Reinfection represents the primary reason for recurrent UTI in most women. In men, recurrence is usually caused by persistence, rather than reinfection, because the source of the repeat infection lies within the urinary tract.

Diagnosis

Chronic bacterial prostatitis is the most common cause of recurrent UTI in men. Commonly, an older man will have dysuria and bacteriuria that recurs after short-term antibiotic therapy. Examination frequently shows not only bacteriuria but also bacteria and white blood cells in expressed prostatic secretions. The patient usually is then presumptively treated with long-term antibiotics. Absence of prostatic inflammation would lead to further work-up for a source of chronic infection, with diagnostic differentials including obstruction and benign prostatic hyperplasia (BPH), bladder stones, or UTI.

Although treatment of chronic prostatitis is frequently initiated based on appearance of prostatic secretions, it is sometimes necessary to perform bacteriologic localization cultures to identify the organism involved and rule out the urethra as a source of infection. This can be done by sequentially collecting the initial voided urine as a urethral sample, midstream urine as a bladder sample, and expressed prostatic secretions and postmassage urine as prostatic samples (Fig. 4–1). Bacterial colony counts in the prostatic specimens far exceed those in the initial voided samples in the case of prostatitis.

Treatment

Successful treatment of recurrent UTI caused by chronic bacterial prostatitis is notoriously difficult in men. This is not because of the organism being treated (usually *E. coli*) but because of the difficulty of sustaining high concentrations of drug within prostatic secretions.

Studies have shown that lipid-soluble antibiotics that are minimally bound to plasma proteins and have favorable dissociation constants diffuse best into the prostate and accumulate to effective levels in the prostatic secretions. Problems arise, however, because of the alkaline nature of infected prostatic secretions and its effect on the pharmacokinetics of many drugs.

Trimethoprim-sulfamethoxazole diffuses well into the prostate. Short-term courses can temporarily clear recurrent UTI associated with prostatitis. However, long-term courses are needed to penetrate the prostate and achieve cures. Three- to six-month courses sterilize the secretions in about one-third of documented cases.

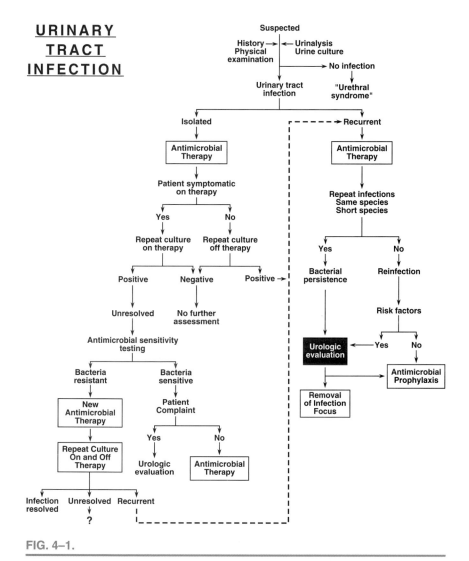

FIG. 4–1.

Segmented culture technique for localizing urinary infections to the urethra or the prostate in men. From Meares EM, Stamey TA: Bacteriologic localization patterns in bacterial prostatitis and urethritis. *Invest Urol* 5:492–518, 1968.

The newer quinolone antibiotics achieve favorable levels within the prostatic secretions. It is likely that they, along with other new oral agents, will produce results as good if not better than those seen with the older drugs. It is unlikely, however, that short-term courses of any oral agent will cure recurrent UTI associated with chronic prostatitis.

RECURRENT URINARY TRACT INFECTION IN CHILDREN

UTI does occur in children, in as many as 5% of girls and 1% to 2% of boys. Foreskins colonized with gram-negative bacteria are responsible for increased rates of infection among neonatal boys, and short urethral length and perineal colonization with fecal flora account for increased rates among girls after the neonatal period. Like pregnant women, children younger than five years of age represent a high-risk group for morbidity associated with UTI, namely in the form of renal scarring, and therefore merit treatment of bacteriuria regardless of symptoms. In addition, radiologic work-up consisting of voiding cystourethrography and renal ultrasonography is liberally performed in most children with first-time UTI. These methods usually identify children with anatomic problems, such as vesicoureteral reflux, that may eventually require surgical intervention.

As many as 80% of children with uncomplicated, lower UTI experience recurrences. It is becoming increasingly apparent that children with UTI not associated with a structural anomaly frequently have some form of voiding dysfunction as the cause for their infection. In children with reflux, voiding dysfunction (if not recognized) can predispose to breakthrough UTI and failure of therapy.

Diagnosis

Voiding dysfunction often is diagnosed by a careful history of voiding habits or by uroflowmetry and sometimes by more complex urodynamic studies. Infrequent voiding ($\leq$ 2 voids/day), straining to void, and poor relaxation of the urethral sphincter muscle can all lead to voiding dysfunction. Voiding frequency, urinary urgency, incontinence, and burning on urination are important features of a voiding history. Sequelae of severe dysfunction are seen on voiding cystourethrography.

Treatment

Treatment of voiding dysfunction consists of a regulated voiding regimen to achieve more complete bladder emptying and oftentimes anticholinergic medication to lower the elevated intravesical pressures. Antibiotic prophylaxis for recurrent UTI in children should be undertaken only after anatomic problems and voiding dysfunction have been either excluded or diagnosed and treated. In addition, the physician should lean toward alternating or interrupting long treatment courses in children rather than using a single agent continuously for years.

The two drugs used most commonly in this role are trimethoprim-sulfamethoxazole and nitrofurantoin. These drugs are generally safe and effective in children. Many physicians recommend an initial two- to four-month period of therapy followed by a period of observation with no medication. If infection recurs, prophylaxis after treatment should consist of the alternate drug for six months. A recent paper established the safety and efficacy of using both drugs as "double prophylaxis" in girls with voiding dysfunction or reflux who experienced breakthrough UTI during single-agent therapy.

Suggested Reading

Johnson MA: Urinary tract infections in women, *Am Family Physician* 41(2):565–571, 1990.

Pfau A, Sacks TG: Effective postcoital quinolone prophylaxis of recurrent urinary tract infections in women, *J Urol* 152:136–138, 1994.

Pfau A, Sacks TG: Effective prophylaxis for recurrent urinary tract infections during pregnancy, *Clin Infect Dis* 14:810–814, 1992.

Pfau A, Sacks TG, Engelstein D: Recurrent urinary tract infections in premenopausal women: Prophylaxis based on an understanding of the pathogenesis, *J Urol* 129: 1153–1157, 1983.

Raz R, Stamm WE: A controlled trial of intravaginal estriol in postmenopausal women with recurrent urinary tract infections, *N Engl J Med* 329:753–756, 1993.

Schaeffer AJ: Infections of the urinary tract, in Walsh PC and others (eds): *Campbell's Urology,* ed 6. Philadelphia, WB Saunders, 1994, pp 731–822.

Smith EM, Elder JS: Double antimicrobial prophylaxis in girls with breakthrough urinary tract infections, *Urology* 43:708–713, 1994.

Stapleton A and others: Postcoital antimicrobial prophylaxis for recurrent urinary tract infection, *JAMA* 264:703–706, 1990.

Strom BL and others: Sexual activity, contraceptive use, and other risk factors for symptomatic and asymptomatic bacteriuria, *Ann Intern Med* 107:816–823 1987.

Uehling DT and others: Phase I clinical trial of vaginal mucosal immunization for recurrent urinary tract infection, *J Urol* 152: 2308–2311, 1994.

5

Urinary Incontinence in Women

More than 20 million Americans suffer from involuntary loss of urine, and the number of individuals with this problem is rising in accord with an aging population. Recent surveys reveal that the incidence of incontinence is greater than 30% of women older than 60 years of age. Diapers for adults have become a $1 billion industry. Increasing numbers of women are requesting evaluation and treatment for incontinence, and the primary-care physician is now confronted with providing not only an accurate diagnosis but a list of treatment options as well. This chapter reviews the definition of urinary incontinence, common classification schemes, patient history and physical examination, voiding diaries, clinical testing, and treatment options.

DEFINITION

The term *urinary incontinence,* strictly interpreted, is the involuntary loss of urine through the urethral meatus. This definition does not, however, include other causes for involuntary urine leakage, such as vesicovaginal fistula or ureteral ectopia.

CLASSIFICATION

Symptomatic classification schemes instead of anatomic terms provide the most accurate means to evaluate incontinent women. There are three principal types of incontinence to be discerned by a careful history: stress, urge, and total.

Stress Incontinence

The sudden loss of urine resulting from actions that increase intraabdominal pressure is known as stress incontinence. Coughing, lifting, sneezing, and laughing are common occurrences known to induce stress incontinence. A current theory proposes that the abdominal pressure transmitted to the bladder is not counteracted by an equal pressure transmitted to the urethra because the bladder neck and urethra have herniated through weakened pelvic structures. Fig. 5–1 illustrates the normal and abnormal anatomy (loss of pelvic support) associated with stress incontinence.

Urge Incontinence

Urge incontinence is defined as a sudden urge to void accompanied by urine loss; such incontinence is associated with variable success at controlling the degree of incontinence. The quantity of lost urine may range from a teaspoonful to the entire contents of the bladder. The volume of urine in the bladder does not

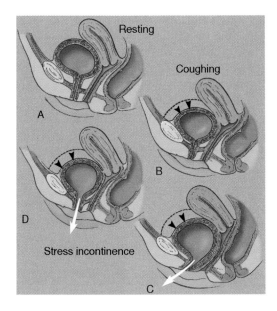

Resting

Coughing

A

B

D

Stress incontinence

C

FIG. 5–1.
A, Bladder and urethra in normal position. **B,** Intraabdominal pressure transmitted to the bladder. **C,** Bladder and urethra in abnormal position with loss of support (hypermobile). **D,** Loss of urethral closure.

dictate when the sudden urge may occur, and patients often notice that small amounts of urine cause urgency. If they are able to hold the urine back, they are perplexed by the small amount of voided urine and the frequent sense that they need to void again after only a short period has passed.

Total Incontinence

Total incontinence is the complete inability to hold urine in the bladder—the patient is constantly wet regardless of efforts to hold the urine. Significant diaper use, both day and night, is common with total incontinence. A nonfunctional urethra usually is found with simple testing (Fig. 5–1*D*).

HISTORY AND PHYSICAL EXAMINATION

The history and physical examination are the most important components of the evaluation of incontinence in women. The history begins with questions about the duration and degree of incontinence and previous surgery to correct stress incontinence. The goal is to identify reversible factors in the patient's behavior or environment and learn of any underlying medical or neurologic disease contributing to the incontinence. It has been reported that up to 50% of incidents of incontinence that occur in hospitalized elderly patients is transient and reverses with recovery and discharge from the hospital. Particular attention should be paid to the onset and type of incontinence (i.e., stress, urge, total, mixed), the position of the patient when it occurs, associated symptoms, nocturnal frequency, and management of the incontinence (i.e., whether the patient uses pads, diapers, or a catheter).

Up to 60% of women have mixed symptoms of urgency and stress-related incontinence, and approximately 30% surveyed have reported urgency alone as the cause of incontinence. The perception of bladder sensation, pelvic prolapse ("heaviness" in the vagina or a bulge), vaginal discharge, or symptoms of estrogen deficiency (dryness and itching) are important signs and symptoms that should be discussed during the history. A careful gynecologic history should include information about operations, parity, infection, trauma, and radiotherapy. Other relevant questions concern previous pelvic trauma, back surgery, medications, sexual and bowel habits, and any concurrent medical disorders.

A voiding diary is essential for quantifying and documenting the amount of lost urine. The diary should record fluid intake and urine output, urgency, time of urine loss, and any physical activity associated with episodes of incontinence. The voiding diary provides a very useful means of involving patients in their care and of uncovering exaggerations when the clinical history is inconsistent with objective testing.

The physical examination must be thorough and not focused entirely on the bladder and urethra. The patient's mental and physical ability can be assessed during the examination. Functional status may play an important role in an elderly patient's physical ability to get to the toilet in time to avoid incontinence. The abdomen should be inspected and palpated for surgical scars, any abnormal masses or lesions, or a distended bladder. A basic neurologic examination should focus on the sensory and motor innervation of the lower urinary tract. Motor and sensory nerves to the bladder and urethral sphincter come from the sacral spinal cord (S-2 to S-4). Sensory dermatome testing of the perineum and motor testing of voluntary anal sphincter contraction and the bulbocavernosus reflex are important steps in the physical examination. The bulbocavernosus reflex is absent in 20% of neurologically intact women. The back and spine should be inspected for scars or asymmetry, and lower extremity reflexes and sensation must be routinely tested.

A systematic pelvic examination is necessary, and the examination is conducted as follows. The patient voids prior to the examination. The status of the vaginal epithelium is ascertained by examining for signs of atrophic vaginitis (i.e., skin that is shiny, dry, smooth, and thin). Some cases of stress incontinence in elderly women can be managed with estrogen replacement alone. The position and appearance of the urethral meatus should be documented. An open and patulous meatus may indicate the presence of a nonfunctional urethra.

One half of a Grave's speculum is used for the pelvic examination. First, the blade is placed against the rectum and the anterior vaginal wall is inspected at rest, with a cough, and with a Valsalva maneuver. The blade is then rotated and the posterior vaginal wall is observed at rest and with stress maneuvers. The cervix is inspected, and the support and position of the uterus are noted. If the patient has previously undergone a hysterectomy, the position and stability of the vaginal cuff are examined, again at rest and with stress maneuvers. A careful examination detects pelvic prolapse of the anterior vaginal wall (cystocele), hypermobility of the proximal urethra, uterine prolapse into the vagina, vaginal vault prolapse after a hysterectomy, herniation of the peritoneum between the uterosacral ligaments (enterocele), or rectal bulging into the vagina (rectocele). Subtle defects can be clarified by repeating the examination with the patient in a standing position.

A 14-French red-rubber catheter is placed in the bladder, and residual urine is measured. A 60-cc syringe without the plunger is connected to the catheter, and the bladder is filled slowly with sterile water. This has been referred to as "eyeball urodynamics." The volume at first sensation of filling, sense of fullness, and urge to void are recorded. Once the bladder is full, the catheter is removed and the stress maneuvers are repeated to demonstrate movement (hypermobility) of the urethra and herniation of the bladder into the vagina (cystocele).

Table 5–1 illustrates a common classification scheme used by urologists to characterize the type of stress incontinence found on physical examination. It is important to note whether leakage occurs immediately with the episodic increases in abdominal pressure. A cough can induce a bladder contraction (bladder instability) when there is a short delay between the cough and the loss of urine. This can lead to a false-positive result inconsistent with genuine stress incontinence. If no leakage is detected with the patient in the lithotomy position,

TABLE 5–1.

Classification of Stress Urinary Incontinence

Type	Characteristics
0	Urethral hypermobility on physical exam with stress but without documented urine loss despite provocative testing
I	Urethral hypermobility on physical exam with documented urine loss, but without cystocele formation
II	Same as in type I, but with cystocele formation
IIA	SUI with cystocele inside vagina
IIB	SUI with cystocele outside vagina
III (proximal sphincter insufficiency)	Intrinsic urethral insufficiency. Urethral support not a factor; usually severe incontinence

she should stand and repeat the stress maneuvers. A history of stress incontinence without objective demonstration of urine loss should prompt referral of the patient for further testing before a diagnosis of stress incontinence is made.

LABORATORY TESTING

Urinalysis, urine culture and sensitivity, and urine cytology should be used to exclude infection or malignancy (for example, carcinoma *in situ*) as a cause of urinary incontinence. A urinary tract infection must be treated before the physician undertakes any instrumentation (cystoscopy or urodynamics) of the bladder or urethra. Serum creatinine is an indicator of renal function in patients with high postvoid residual urine volumes or severe cystocele. These disorders may cause the ureters to become obstructed due to herniation of the bladder through the pelvic floor and introitus.

Cystoscopy is used to evaluate the bladder for pain with filling, hypermobility with straining, site of urinary obstruction, obstructed urinary flow, and total incontinence with an open-appearing and patulous proximal urethra. A history of hematuria or finding of red blood cells on urinalysis requires cystoscopic examination to exclude a bladder tumor, stone, or foreign body.

Radiographic studies are used to evaluate the possibility of type III stress urinary incontinence (an open bladder neck at rest or leakage with minimal abdominal pressure on the bladder) or moderate to severe pelvic prolapse. Radiography is also used to obtain information related to obstruction of the urethra, resulting from previous surgery for incontinence (Fig. 5–2). The voiding cystourethrogram (VCUG) under fluoroscopic control is used to examine the blad-

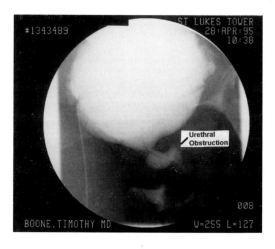

FIG. 5–2.

Radiograph of urethral obstruction on voiding cystourethrogram following needle suspension.

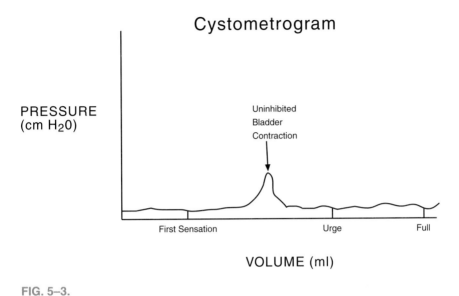

Cystometrogram

PRESSURE
(cm H$_2$0)

Uninhibited
Bladder
Contraction

First Sensation   Urge   Full

VOLUME (ml)

FIG. 5–3.

Cystometrogram demonstrating the volumes at first sensation, urgency, and fullness. An uninhibited bladder contraction is seen midway through filling the bladder.

der filled with radiographic contrast while the patient stands, strains, coughs, and voids. The VCUG also gives information about reflux into the ureters; and, if present, urethral diverticula as well as a contrast image showing postvoid residual urine. The bladder neck will open with a sudden bladder contraction, and because a fluoroscopic image cannot distinguish between an anatomically incompetent proximal urethra (bladder neck) and a sudden bladder contraction, a small pressure catheter is often placed in the bladder during the study. Both the pressure in the bladder and the VCUG images are recorded together. This joint modality is known as videourodynamics. Simple urodynamic studies are used to help the clinician improve the accuracy of the diagnosis and select the proper management technique for urinary incontinence. The diagnosis of urinary incontinence with urodynamic testing requires that the incontinence be reproduced during the test. A filling cystometrogram (CMG) records the pressure within the bladder while the bladder is being filled at a set rate, usually 40 to 60 milliliters per minute. The volume at first sensation of filling, first urge to void, and capacity are recorded and marked on the CMG (Fig. 5–3). Sudden bladder contractions that occur as the patient attempts to hold her urine are seen as pressure waves on the CMG and referred to as involuntary bladder contractions, with or without the sensation of urgency or incontinence. When the sudden sensation of urgency is associated with an involuntary contraction on the CMG and incontinence is documented, the patient has urge incontinence secondary to involuntary bladder contractions (i.e., detrusor instability). Hand washing, the sound of running water, or heel bouncing may precipitate urge incontinence in the laboratory.

The adult bladder holds 400 to 600 milliliters of urine and has a pressure of less than 12 cm H_2O at capacity. A slow, steady rise in pressure with filling demonstrates poor compliance of the bladder wall (fibrosis), which is commonly seen after radiation therapy to the pelvis for gynecologic malignancy or damage to the peripheral nerve supply of the bladder. The normal, anatomically supported urethra closes with increases in abdominal pressure. A urethra that has been damaged by radiotherapy, trauma, multiple operations, or nerve injury does not close with abdominal pressure (Valsalva pressure recorded on the CMG). The urethra also appears well supported but open with straining viewed on VCUG or during the pelvic examination.

OPTIONS FOR TREATMENT OF STRESS INCONTINENCE

Pelvic exercises, medication, bladder training, vaginal pessaries, electrical stimulation, and surgery represent the broad treatment categories available to the clinician once the diagnosis of stress incontinence has been made. Table 5–2 shows the relative success rates with several common treatment options.

Pelvic floor or "Kegel" exercises have a reported cure rate up to 70% in several surveys. Pelvic floor exercises, when properly done, strengthen the levator ani muscles; these muscles form a supporting hammock elevating the pelvic organs, including the bladder and urethra. Thoroughly educating patients is the key to effective pelvic floor exercises. Women must be taught which muscles to contract and be informed about the duration and frequency of contractions that are most beneficial—a simple instruction sheet is inadequate to properly educate incontinent patients. At the time of pelvic examination, the physician places two fingers in the patient's vagina and places the other hand on her abdomen. The patient is asked to contract her muscles as if she were stopping urination, and the physician notes the isolation of the pelvic floor musculature without abdominal muscle tightening. The pelvic floor contraction/relaxation exercises are done to the "count of four" for each contraction for five minutes at least twice daily.

Biofeedback techniques and other instruments measuring contraction pressure serve to visually reinforce the "Kegel" method. Weighted vaginal cones help women identify the proper muscles to contract in order to retain the cone. Weighted cones can be worn for 15 minutes twice daily while walking or standing. Electrical stimulation to the pelvic floor musculature through a vaginal probe has been used to further reinforce isolation and exercise of the proper muscles. The ideal parameters for stimulation and treatment duration are still under investigation.

Estrogen preparations and alpha-adrenergic agonists are the principal medications used to control stress incontinence. Smooth muscle in the bladder base and proximal urethra is stimulated to contract with alpha-adrenergic agents to help with urethral closure during stress maneuvers. Phenylpropanolamine is most commonly used and is found in many over-the-counter cold preparations (Ornade® Spansule®—SmithKline Beecham Pharmaceuticals, Entex® LA—Procter & Gamble Pharmaceuticals, and Tavist-D®—Sandoz Consumer). Estrogen replacement in postmenopausal women thickens the mucosal lining of the urethra and vagina. Estrogen is believed to improve the mucosal seal in the urethra as the walls coapt toward the lumen with transmitted abdominal pressure.

Traditionally, bladder training has been used to control urinary urgency and urge incontinence. By studying the voiding diary, the clinician assigns a set voiding interval, often referred to as timed voiding. If the patient voids every hour, the timed voiding interval is set at 45 minutes. She is instructed to void only at the assigned times. Each week, the timed interval is increased by 15 minutes;

TABLE 5–2.
Outcome of stress incontinence treatments

	Treatment Options				
	Behavioral technique			Surgical technique	
Outcome	Pelvic muscle exercise	Bladder training	Pharmacologic: Alpha agonist	Retropubic suspension	Needle suspension
Percent cured	12	16	0–14	78	84
Percent improved	75	54	19–60	5	4
Total percent	87	70	19–74	83	88
Percent side effects	None		Minimal to 20	–	
Percent complications	None		5–33	20	

From Urinary Incontinence Guideline Panel: Urinary Incontinence in Adults: Clinical Practice Guideline. AHCPR Pub. No. 92-0038. Rockville, MD, Department of Health and Human Services, p58, 1992. Modified with permission.

eventually, urgency is controlled by reinforcing cortical control over the bladder's sensory mechanism. A few studies have shown equal effectiveness with stress incontinence. Combined with pelvic floor exercises, bladder training is an excellent first-line treatment for 40-year-old women with new-onset stress incontinence mixed with occasional urgency symptoms.

Vaginal pessaries and diaphragms have been used to control stress incontinence. These objects provide bladder base support and prevent hypermobility of the bladder neck and urethra with sudden increases in abdominal pressure. Difficulty in placement and discomfort have limited the role of such devices in controlling incontinence. Early experience with the Hodge pessary has been good, but long-term effectiveness has not been established.

Surgical options should be discussed if it is clear that genuine stress incontinence is present and conservative measures have failed to control urine loss. There are six major categories representing more than 100 surgical procedures that have been developed to cure stress incontinence (Table 5–3). The choice of surgical procedure is based on the following criteria: the patient's motivation to gain continence, whether the procedure is a primary or recurrent operation, presence of pelvic prolapse, integrity of the proximal urethral sphincter, concomitant abdominal or pelvic pathology, and the degree of urethrovesical junction hypermobility. Procedural cure rates versus cure rates with conservative measures should be discussed (Table 5–2).

TABLE 5–3.

**Surgical Treatment of
Stress Incontinence**

Anterior Colporrhaphy
  With or without Kelly plication
Abdominal Retropubic Urethropexy
  Marshall-Marchetti-Krantz
  Burch operation
  Paravaginal repair
  Lapides procedure
Transvaginal Needle Suspension
  Pereyra
  Stamey
  Gittes
  Raz
Pubovaginal Sling
Artificial Urinary Sphincter
Collagen Urethral Implant

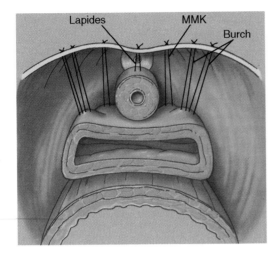

FIG. 5–4.

Operations for retropubic repair: Marshall-Marchetti-Krantz, Burch, Lapides. All serve to support the urethra and prevent downward movement with increases in intraabdominal pressure.

Anterior colporrhaphy is used to reduce and repair a cystocele that has herniated into the anterior vaginal wall. This procedure is associated with a poor long-term outcome for correcting stress incontinence if surgical restoration of proper bladder neck support is not done at the same time. The best long-term outcome has been associated with abdominal retropubic urethropexies (Fig. 5–4). Retropubic procedures are indicated as a primary or secondary treatment for a hypermobile urethra with a functional proximal sphincter and no significant cystocele (i.e., type I stress incontinence).

Pereyra popularized a transvaginal needle procedure in 1959. Numerous modifications have evolved, but the principles of the technique are the same. Surgeons have given their names to their particular modifications (Stamey, Gittes, Raz). The region lateral to the bladder neck on either side is sutured blindly or through a vaginal incision and then supported by transferring the permanent suture threaded on a needle to a suprapubic location where the suspension sutures are tied to the rectus fascia or anchored in the pubic bone. The operative time and recovery period are short in comparison with the abdominal retropubic operations. Some centers perform needle suspensions as outpatient surgery. Long-term outcome data are still being collected to compare the efficacy of needle suspensions to retropubic urethropexies. Type III stress incontinence with an incompetent proximal urethra is treated with a collagen implant, a pubovaginal sling, or an artificial urinary sphincter. Suspension procedures fail in more than 50% of cases when a poor sphincter mechanism is simply supported in a different position. Collagen injected beneath the bladder neck mucosa, a piece of fascia lifting and compressing the urethra, or a mechanical cuff around the proximal urethra (artificial urinary sphincter) are all viable methods of treating type III stress incontinence. The surgeon should discuss the risks and benefits of each option with the patient when she is making a decision regarding operative therapy to correct stress incontinence.

A variety of options exist for the treatment of stress incontinence. A careful history and physical examination, along with simple diagnostic testing, leads to an accurate diagnosis. Conservative methods should be explained and tried before surgery is undertaken—morbidity is greater with operative therapy and long-term data regarding efficacy are still being collected. Patients who are refractory to oral medication but are deemed medically unfit for surgery may become catheter-dependent. Monthly catheter changes reduce infections, and a closed collection system must be used to maintain a bacteria-free environment.

The primary-care physician should be able to document and demonstrate stress incontinence. When the clinical history and examination clearly show urinary incontinence with stress maneuvers, the physician should be able to offer instruction in pelvic floor exercises and prescribe oral medications that may help control the problem. A history of urge incontinence and lack of urine loss with stress maneuvers during the examination should guide the primary-care physician to rule out infection or carcinoma *in situ*. Persistent symptoms without infection warrant referral to the urologist. Failure to control stress incontinence with exercises or pharmacotherapy at the primary-care level justifies referral to the urologist for consideration of surgical therapy.

OPTIONS FOR TREATMENT OF URGE INCONTINENCE

The inability to postpone urination when a sudden urge to void occurs is called urge incontinence. Urge incontinence may be caused by a neurologic disorder (multiple sclerosis, spinal cord injury, cerebrovascular accident, or urinary tract infection) or may be idiopathic in origin. Most cases of urge incontinence and detrusor instability have no identifiable neurologic etiology. Aging bladder muscle is prone to the development of unstable or poorly controlled contractions. Anticholinergic and antispasmodic agents have been used to help prevent or delay sudden bladder contractions leading to urge incontinence. Oxybutynin (Ditropan®—Marion Merrill Dow), propantheline bromide (Pro-BanthAne®—Roberts), and hyoscyamine sulfate (Levsin®—Schwarz Pharmaceuticals) are the most common oral preparations used to treat urge incontinence.

SELECTED READING

1. Horbach NS: Genuine stress urinary incontinence: best surgical approach, *Contemp Obstet Gynecol* 37:53–61, 1992.
2. McGuire EJ: Pathophysiology of incontinence in elderly women, in O'Donnell P (ed): *Geriatric Urology.* Boston, Little-Brown, 1994, pp 221–227.

3. Nygaard I: Nonsurgical therapy for stress urinary incontinence, *Contemp Obstet Gynecol* 38: 79–91, 1993.
4. Resnick NM, Yalla SV: Evaluation and medical management of urinary incontinence, in Walsh PC and others (eds): *Campbell's Urology,* ed 6. Philadelphia, WB Saunders, 1992, pp 643–658.
5. Snyder JA, Lipsitz DU: Evaluation of female urinary incontinence, *Urol Clin North Am* 18:197–209, 1991.

6

Nonmalignant Diseases of the Prostate

While controversy rages regarding the public health issues and the economic impact of early detection and treatment strategies for prostate cancer, benign disorders of the prostate gland, including benign prostatic hyperplasia (BPH) and prostatitis, quietly account for more than 3.5 million physician visits per year, as compared with fewer than 1 million attributable to prostate cancer. The clinician must have the knowledge to systematically evaluate patients suffering from these disorders because of their complex nature. For example, symptoms of chronic prostatitis can be vexing for both patient and doctor, yet only a small proportion of these patients have a documentable bacterial infection that can be cured with appropriate antibiotics. Understanding how to identify such patients is essential to avoiding the frustration of needless and ineffective long courses of antibiotics in patients unlikely to benefit from them.

BPH was once thought to be a relatively simple disease process of obstruction of the lower urinary tract due to prostatic enlargement. Historically, there was only a single therapeutic option: prostatectomy, either transurethral or open. However, in the past decade, our understanding of BPH has evolved to the extent that it is now rightly viewed as a highly complex disease with an uncertain etiology and natural history. The myriad of potential therapies range from "watchful waiting," to medical therapy with α-blockers or 5-α reductase inhibitors, to more invasive therapies using heat, microwave, electrovaporization, laser technology, balloon dilatation, and prosthetic stents as well as the more traditional approach, prostatectomy. All of these therapies may be used to relieve symptoms.

Even among urologists, there is still strong disagreement regarding the need for invasive diagnostic tests, specifically urodynamics, in evaluation of patients with BPH as well as regarding the use of such techniques in the selection and monitoring of appropriate therapy. A basic understanding of important nonmalignant prostatic diseases helps general practitioners distinguish patients who can be managed safely and effectively from those who may require more expert evaluation and management.

BACKGROUND: PROSTATIC ANATOMY AND PHYSIOLOGY

The prostate has three major glandular regions or "zones," which were first described by McNeal in 1968. These regions differ histologically and biologically and exhibit differing predispositions toward the disease processes that commonly occur within the prostate (i.e., prostate cancer, prostatitis, and BPH) (Fig. 6–1, Table 6–1). The rapid integration of transrectal ultrasonography into the routine practice of urology has led to a resurgence of interest in the zonal anatomy of the prostate because, for the first time, these zones have become clearly "visible" to the clinician. Notably, BPH occurs almost exclusively in the

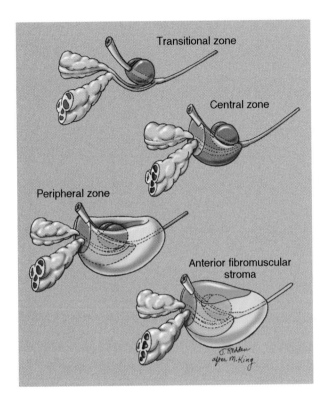

FIG. 6–1.

Zonal anatomy of the prostate. There are three glandular zones and the anterior fibromuscular stroma. In the prostate of young adults, the transition zone comprises 5%, the central zone 25%, and the peripheral zone 70%. The transition zone is the site of origin of benign prostatic hyperplasia. In men older than 50 years of age, the transition zone may comprise a large proportion of the glandular prostatic tissue in marked benign prostatic hyperplasia. (From Greene DR and others: Relationship between clinical stage and histological zone of origin in early prostate cancer: morphometric analysis, *Br J Urol* 68:499–509, 1991. Reproduced with permission.)

transition zone and periurethral region. In men with severe BPH, the transition zone, which typically makes up only 5% of the volume of the normal 20-gram prostate, can grow to more than 100 grams, compressing the remaining zones of the prostate around it. About 25% of all prostate cancers arise within the transition zone, which is far from the examining finger during a digital rectal exami-

TABLE 6–1.

Zonal anatomy of the prostate: Histological, Biological, and Clinico-Pathological Distributions

	Central Zone	Transition Zone	Peripheral Zone
Volume of normal prostates	25%	5%	70%
Anatomic Landmarks			
Intraprostatic relationships	Ejaculatory ducts	Surrounds prox urethra	Distal prostatic urethra
Adjacent structures	Seminal vesicles	Bladder neck	Rectum
Urethral orifices of ducts	Verumontanum, adjacent to ejac, ducts	Posterolateral wall of prostatic urethra proximal to verumontanum	Posterolateral wall of prostatic urethra distal to verumontanum
Histologic Features			
Epithelium	Complex, large polygonal glands with intraluminal ridges	Simple, small rounded glands	Simple, small rounded glands
Stroma	Compact	Compact	Loose
Proposed embryonic origin	Wolffian duct	Urogenital sinus	Urogenital sinus
Tissue Sampling Technique			
Transurethral resection	Poor	Good	Poor
Needle biopsy (TRUS)	Variable	Poor	Good
Involvement with pathologic process			
Atrophy	Infrequent	Variable	Frequent

nation and is difficult to visualize clearly with transrectal ultrasonography. It is adequately sampled, however, during a standard transurethral resection of the prostate.

The remaining 75% of cancers arise within the peripheral zone, which is in proximity to the examining finger during a digital rectal examination and is well visualized during transrectal ultrasonography. Prostatitis and glandular atrophy, two other common pathologic processes of the prostate gland, are also typically located within the peripheral zone, perhaps because the ductal anatomy of this zone predisposes it to reflux of intraurethral urine to a greater extent than other zones. This region is extremely difficult to resect during a transurethral prostatectomy because it lies in a predominantly distal direction to the verumontanum and is close to the striated urethral sphincter.

The central zone, which makes up 25% of the normal prostate gland, is rarely involved in any of these pathologic processes. Currently, an understanding of the zonal relationships of the prostate remains an important tool for clinical management of prostate diseases.

Benign Prostatic Hyperplasia

BPH is a pathologic process characterized by enlargement of the prostate gland. The disorder can be recognized grossly and microscopically using well-defined pathologic criteria. While the terms are used synonymously, *benign prostatic hyperplasia* technically is distinct from the clinical disease termed *prostatism*, which has a constellation of symptoms that often are associated with and attributed to BPH. BPH gradually occurs in the aging male population and is widely prevalent. Autopsy studies have demonstrated that approximately 50% of men have histologic evidence of BPH by the age of 60, and this rises to 80% of men by the age of 80.

The process of BPH, rather than being a diffuse hyperplastic enlargement of the entire prostate, follows a well-characterized progression of events. The process begins with formation of periurethral and transition zone stromal nodules, followed by convergent epithelial ingrowth and budding and branching morphogenesis within micronodules, and lastly by diffuse enlargement of these "benign prostatic hyperplasia nodules."

While the pathologic morphology and progression of BPH have been clearly defined, relatively little is known about the etiology of BPH except that it requires the presence of functioning testes and correlates closely with aging. Epidemiologic studies searching for an association between BPH and diet, smoking, caffeine, frequency of sexual intercourse, medications, vasectomy, or other diseases have been negative.

As mentioned, BPH is associated with prostatism, which is a symptom complex that comprises both obstructive and irritative components. However, while 70% of males will develop histologic evidence of BPH by the age of 70, only 20% to 25% of males will undergo prostatectomy for BPH by this age, suggesting that the onset and severity of symptoms associated with prostatism do not correlate completely with the pathologic process of BPH. For example, while increasing prostate size generally correlates with objective parameters of bladder outlet obstruction, several studies have failed to correlate the extent of prostate enlargement with the severity of prostatism or the magnitude of bladder outlet obstruction. Thus, clinical diagnosis of BPH is made only after a thorough history and physical examination along with several objective measurements of lower urinary tract function.

A number of scoring systems (e.g., Madsen-Iversen, Boyarsky, and most recently the American Urological Association [AUA] Symptom Index) (Fig. 6–2) have been developed to quantify the type and degree of symptoms experienced by men with BPH. The AUA Symptom Index is a validated, self-administered list of seven questions regarding various symptoms typically associated with BPH. Each question has a possible response on an increasing scale of 0 (never experienced) to 5 (experienced all the time), with a maximum total score of 35. These questionnaires are useful in making therapeutic choices for patients according to the severity of disease as well as for monitoring the response to therapy. However, it should be emphasized that high scores on these questionnaires are not diagnostic of BPH—no combination of symptoms is specific for this disease process alone. Based on the AUA Symptom Index, where a score of 8 or greater indicates moderate symptoms, approximately 25% of men older than 50 years of age experience symptoms of BPH. The available literature on the natural history of BPH suggests that the clinical course is variable rather than progressive. Many patients with BPH, especially those with mild symptoms, improve without treatment, although it is impossible to predict which patients will improve spontaneously.

An initial evaluation for BPH should include a detailed medical history focusing on the urinary tract as well as the general health of the patient. Physical examination should include a digital rectal examination and a focused neurologic examination. Such examination establishes the approximate size of the prostate and uncovers neurologic problems that might be causing symptoms. If the digital rectal examination reveals any abnormality, especially induration or the presence of a nodule, the patient should be referred to a urologist. Screening studies demonstrate that 25% to 30% of asymptomatic men with an abnormal digital rectal examination or prostate-specific antigen have detectable prostate cancer; in men with symptoms, the frequency of prostate cancer is higher. Urinalysis is performed to rule out a urinary tract infection or microscopic hematuria, which also would require referral for further evaluation. Analysis of serum creatine as a gross assessment of renal function should be performed, and elevation should prompt the appropriate imaging studies to evaluate the upper urinary tract. While measurement of serum prostate-specific antigen is considered by some to be an optional test for men with prostatism, I believe strongly that this measurement should be part of the evaluation for men older than 50 years of age as a screening evaluation for prostate cancer, regardless of symptoms. The AUA Symptom Index should be obtained, and the patient's symptoms should be classified as mild (0 to 7), moderate (8 to 19), or severe (20 to 35). *The symptom score should be the primary determinant of treatment response and disease progression in the follow-up period.*

Patients with a normal initial evaluation and symptoms considered mild on the basis of the AUA Symptom Index assessment do not need further diagnostic

International Prostate Symptom Score (I-PSS)

Patient name:	Not at all	Less than 1 time in 5	Less than half the time	About half the time	More than half the time	Almost always	Your score
1. Incomplete emptying Over the past month, how often have you had a sensation of not emptying your bladder completely after you finished urinating?	0	1	2	3	4	5	
2. Frequency Over the past month, how often have you had to urinate again less than two hours after you finished urinating?	0	1	2	3	4	5	
3. Intermittency Over the past month, how often have you found you stopped and started again several times when you urinated?	0	1	2	3	4	5	
4. Urgency Over the past month, how often have you found it difficult to postpone urination?	0	1	2	3	4	5	
5. Weak stream Over the past month, how often have you had a weak urinary stream?	0	1	2	3	4	5	
6. Straining Over the past month, how often have you had to push or strain to begin urination?	0	1	2	3	4	5	

	None	1 time	2 times	3 times	4 times	5 or more times	
7. Nocturia Over the past month, how many times did you most typically get up to urinate from the time you went to bed at night until the time you got up in the morning?	0	1	2	3	4	5	
Total I-PSS Score=							

Quality of Life due to Urinary Symptoms	Delighted	Pleased	Mostly satisfied	Mixed-about equally satisfied and dissatisfied	Mostly dissatisfied	Unhappy	Terrible
If you were to spend the rest of your life with your urinary condition just the way it is now, how would you feel about that?	0	1	2	3	4	5	6

The International Prostate Symptom Score (I-PSS) is based on the answers to seven questions concerning urinary symptoms.

Each question allows the patient to choose one out of five answers indicating increasing severity of the particular symptom.

The answers are assigned points from 0 to 5. The total score can therefore range from 0 to 35 (asymptomatic to very symptomatic).

Furthermore, the International Consensus Committee (ICC) recommends the use of only a single question to assess the quality of life. The answers to this question range from "delighted" to "terrible" or 0 to 6. Although this single question may or may not capture the global impact of BPH symptoms or quality of life, it may serve as a valuable starting point for a doctor-patient conversation.

The ICC strongly recommends that all physicians who counsel patients suffering from symptoms of prostatism utilize these measures not only during the initial interview but also during and after treatment in order to monitor treatment response.

The International Consensus Committee (ICC) under the patronage of the World Health Organization (WHO) has agreed to use the symptom index for benign prostatic hyperplasia (BPH), which has been developed by the American Urological Association (AUA) Measurement Committee, as the official worldwide symptoms assessment tool for patients suffering from prostatism.

FIG. 6–2.

American Urological Association Symptom Index. Reproduced with permission.

evaluation and should be placed on a watchful waiting program without treatment. In men with more pronounced symptoms, further evaluation with a urinary flow rate and a postvoid measurement of residual urine is helpful as an objective measure of bladder outlet obstruction. Intravenous pyelogram, urodynamics, and cystourethroscopy are reserved for men with complicating factors (e.g., hematuria, urinary tract infection, or a history of urinary tract surgery).

In standard practice, men with moderate symptoms are often offered a trial of medical therapy with one agent from the two classes of drugs found to be effective for moderate BPH, 5-α reductase inhibitors and α-1 adrenergic receptor blockers. Within the prostate, the enzyme 5α reductase type II converts testosterone to dihydrotestosterone, which is the major mediator of androgen action within the prostate. In men with male pseudohermaphroditism due to 5α reductase type II deficiency, there is a marked reduction of circulating and intraprostatic dihydrotestosterone, but plasma levels of testosterone are normal. At puberty, these males virilize because of the normal pubertal increase in circulating testosterone, but their prostates remain small and never develop BPH. Observation of these events formed the basis for the development of 5α reductase type II inhibitors (e.g., finasteride [Proscar®—Merck & Co., Inc.]), for the treatment of BPH. Data from randomized clinical trials have demonstrated that treatment with 5-mg per day of finasteride led to a 19% decrease in prostate volume compared with placebo and yielded modest improvement in symptoms and maximal urinary flow rates. Alpha-1 adrenergic receptor blockers have a different mechanism of action. These agents presumably block the abundant adrenergic receptors located on the smooth muscle cells of the BPH stroma. In large, randomized, placebo-controlled trials, both α-1 adrenergic receptor blockers have demonstrated at least short-term safety and efficacy over placebo, with modest reductions in symptom severity and modest increases in urinary flow rates. Although medical therapy may reduce symptoms, no data currently prove that medical therapy inhibits progression of BPH or decreases the probability of future prostatectomy.

There are a few well-defined indications for surgical intervention in BPH. However, these indications are experienced by only a small minority of patients suffering from BPH. Surgical treatment is indicated when chronic outflow obstruction has resulted in bladder decompensation, overflow incontinence, or renal impairment. Other indications for prompt surgical intervention include more than one episode of acute urinary retention; multiple urinary tract infections; and, rarely, severe hematuria related to BPH. Relative indications for surgical intervention also include a large postvoid volume of urine. Until recently, prostatectomy represented the only accepted treatment for BPH, but interest is growing in new minimally invasive alternatives, both surgical and nonsurgical, in the management of this disease. While medical therapy is evolving into first-line therapy for men with moderate symptoms, those who fail to respond to medical therapy and those with moderate to severe symptoms are candidates for the more invasive treatments.

PROSTATITIS

In 1980, Stamey wrote that prostatitis was a "wastebasket of clinical ignorance" due to variations in terminology, diagnostic criteria, and treatment. However, a few simple diagnostic criteria and clinical laboratory tests make it possible to separate patients suspected of having prostatitis into one of several disease categories to facilitate initiation of appropriate therapy (Table 6–2). In addition to a good clinical history and physical examination, essential components of the evaluation for prostatitis are bacteriologic localization studies based on a fractionated microscopic examination of urine and expressed prostatic secretions or the four-specimen test, which was first described by Meares and Stamey (Fig. 6–3). In brief, the test is conducted as follows. After appropriate cleansing of the glans penis, the first 10 milliliters of voided urine is collected (VB1), and a second specimen in a separate collection container is collected during midstream voiding (VB2). After the patient has completed voiding, the examiner performs a prostatic massage by inserting a gloved, lubricated finger into the rectum and pressing firmly against the prostate while sweeping several times from base to apex. The penile urethra is then milked by the examiner to express prostatic secretions, which are collected in a third specimen cup or, if the amount is limited, on a clean glass slide. Immediately after the prostatic massage, a final voided urine specimen is obtained (VB3). The diagnosis of prostatic infection is made when the quantitative bacteria colony counts of the expressed prostatic secretions and VB3 significantly exceed those of the urethral (VB1) and bladder (VB2) specimens.

Acute bacterial prostatitis is the most straightforward type of prostatitis to diagnose and treat. The diagnosis of *chronic bacterial prostatitis* is more difficult to establish but is the most common cause of relapsing urinary tract infections in men. Unfortunately, while both entities respond to antibiotic therapy, they occur in fewer than 10% to 20% of men who typically have symptoms suggestive of prostatitis. The overwhelming majority of patients form an ill-defined group that is much less well understood. Clinically, these patients also have a wide variety of symptoms, including pain and discomfort referred to the lower back, genitalia, testicles, perineum, and rectum. Irritative and obstructive symptoms of the lower urinary tract often accompany this clinical picture.

For lack of a better system, these patients are currently classified by examination of expressed prostatic secretions into those with *nonbacterial prostatitis* when the secretions contain increased numbers of white blood cells and lipid-laden macrophages and those with *prostatodynia,* when the findings revealed by the prostatic secretions are unremarkable. However, the significance of these differences remains unproven. Patients with prostatodynia probably have a mixture of non-infectious, noninflammatory pelvic floor and psychosomatic disorders. The diagnosis and treatment of both of these entities can be frustrating for both the clinician and patient, with patients often seeing many physicians and undergoing

TABLE 6–2.
Classification and Clinical Features of Prostatitis

Syndrome	History of confirmed UTI	Abnormal rectal exam?	Excessive WBCs in EPS	Positive culture of EPS or VB3>VB1	Common causative agents	Response to antimicrobials	Approximate clinical incidence
Acute bacterial prostatitis	Yes	Yes	Yes	Yes	Coliform bacteria	Yes	5%–10%
Chronic bacterial prostatitis	±	Yes	Yes	Yes	Coliform bacteria	Yes	5%–10%
Nonbacterial prostatitis	No	±	Yes	No	None, *Chlamydia?* *Ureaplasma?*	Usually not	40%
Prostatodynia	No	No	No	No	None	No	40%
Nosocomial prostatitis	No	Yes	±	Yes	Coliform bacteria	Yes	?
Rare types	±	Yes	±	±	Fungi, Mycobacteria, Parasites	±	?

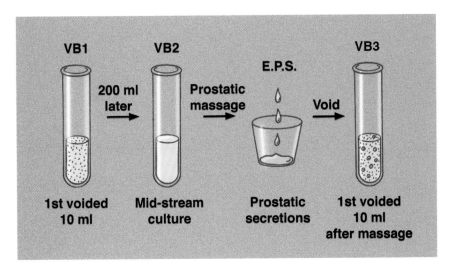

FIG. 6–3.

Bacteriologic localization studies based on fractionated microscopic examination of urine and expressed prostatic secretions (EPS) or the four-specimen test, as first described by Meares and Stamey. (From Meares EM, Stamey TA: Bacteriologic localization patterns in bacterial prostatitis and urethritis, *Invest Urol* 5:492–518, 1968).

innumerable and lengthy courses of antibiotic therapy. Patients undergoing an evaluation for chronic prostatitis should also undergo a voiding flow rate, a postvoid residual (PVR) determination, and a transrectal ultrasound (TRUS) of the prostate. The flow rate and PVR may demonstrate evidence of lower urinary tract obstruction, which is a predisposing risk factor for chronic bacterial prostatitis. TRUS may demonstrate the presence of prostatic calculi, which usually cause no symptoms but can become infected and serve as a source of recurrent urinary tract infection. In some patients, more comprehensive evaluation of voiding physiology with video urodynamics as well as flexible cystoscopy may be indicated.

ACUTE BACTERIAL PROSTATITIS AND PROSTATIC ABSCESSES

Acute bacterial prostatitis typically is manifested in a striking combination of high fever; chills; perineal, suprapubic, or lower back pain; painful bowel movements; urethral discharge; hematuria and obstructive or irritative voiding symptoms; and even frank urinary retention. This clinical manifestation often is preceded by a prodromal syndrome of malaise, fever, arthralgia, or myalgia. On physical examination, the prostate is often exquisitely tender, swollen, warm, and indurated. During acute infection, massage for expressed prostatic secretions and urethral catheterization or other endourologic procedures are contraindicated, as they are likely to cause bacteremic sepsis. However, a simple urine culture often reveals the responsible organism, because these patients are often bacteriuric.

The pathogenesis of acute bacterial prostatitis most likely involves reflux of infected urine into prostatic ducts, an event that may occur during any increase in intraurethral pressure, no matter how transient. Common predisposing risk factors for the development of acute bacterial prostatitis are bladder outlet obstruction (due to stricture, stenosis, calculi, or BPH), poor bladder emptying due to other causes (diabetic cystopathy or spinal cord injury), urinary tract infection, advancing age, instrumentation of the lower urinary tract, and the presence of an indwelling urethral catheter. The most common pathogens identified are *Escherichia coli* (80%), Enterobacteriaceae (10% to 15%), and Enterococci (5% to 10%). Occasionally, such gram-positive organisms as *Staphylococcus epidermidis* may ascend from the anterior urethra and cause acute prostatic infection. The role of sexually transmitted microorganisms, such as *Ureaplasma urealyticum, Chlamydia trachomatis,* and *Trichomonas vaginalis* remains controversial. *Neisseria gonorrhea,* which was a common causative agent for both acute bacterial prostatitis and prostatic abscess in the preantibiotic era, is now rarely seen. Immunosuppressed patients may have prostatic infection due to rare types of infectious agents, including *Mycobacterium tuberculosis,* and fungi, such as *Cryptococcus neoformans* and *Coccidioides immitis.*

The marked inflammation of the prostate gland during acute bacterial prostatitis allows a number of antibiotics to penetrate the prostate. After urine and blood cultures, intravenous therapy with a fluoroquinolone, a combination of an aminoglycoside/beta lactam (ampicillin/gentamicin, ampicillin/tobramycin), or a third-generation cephalosporin should be initiated. Patients with acute urinary retention should have a punch suprapubic cystostomy tube rather than an indwelling urethral catheter placed. After the patient responds with a decrease in symptoms and fever, the patient may be switched within 48 hours to long-term oral therapy for 4 to 16 weeks to prevent relapse or chronic bacterial prostatitis. Some typical regimens include trimethoprim/sulfamethoxazole 160/800 orally twice daily, ciprofloxacin 500 mg orally twice daily, or ofloxacin 300 mg orally twice daily. Patients refractory to primary therapy or those with symptoms that persist for a prolonged period should be suspected of having developed a prostatic abscess.

Prostatic abscesses are relatively rare but can be seen most typically in immunocompromised patients, such as those with AIDS or diabetes. Further imaging studies, including computed tomography, on which abscesses appear as areas of low attenuation within the prostate, and TRUS, on which they appear as hypoechoic areas suspicious for fluid collection, are indicated to confirm the diagnosis. Traditionally, prostatic abscesses have been drained via transurethral "unroofing" but, more recently, transrectal drainage under TRUS guidance has been used. Rarely, perineal drainage or formal resection is required when the abscess is perforated or recurrent.

One week after antibiotic treatment is ended, the patient should be evaluated for eradication of the bacterial infection. In patients with persistent bacteriuria, an additional six-week course, perhaps with a second antibiotic, should be instituted.

CHRONIC BACTERIAL PROSTATITIS, NONBACTERIAL PROSTATITIS, AND PROSTATODYNIA

Chronic bacterial prostatitis, nonbacterial prostatitis, and prostatodynia, unlike acute bacterial prostatitis, present with identical clinical signs and symptoms. Although some men develop chronic bacterial prostatitis after a well-defined bout of acute bacterial prostatitis, in others no such history is found. However, men older than 40 years of age often have a history of recurrent epididymitis. A tender, boggy prostate may be noted on digital rectal examination, but this is not a specific finding. After exclusion of an inflammatory urethral reaction by history and examination of VB1, approximately 10 to 15 polymorphonuclear leukocytes/high-power field in the expressed prostatic secretions is indicative of prostatitis. When VB1 and VB2 are free of leukocytes, 10 or more granulocytes in VB3 is also highly indicative of chronic prostatitis and is comparable to elevated leukocyte numbers in the expressed prostatic secretions. While prostatic secretions may be transiently elevated due to recent ejaculation, a persistent increase in leukocytes in the secretions is most likely due to chronic bacterial prostatitis or nonbacterial prostatitis. Furthermore, on the basis of the four-specimen test, chronic *bacterial* prostatitis is confirmed when there is a 10-fold or higher concentration of urinary pathogens in the VB3 (generally $\geq 10^4$ CFU/ml) than in the VB2.

The hallmark of chronic bacterial prostatitis is relapsing bacteriuria, in which the same pathogen is found repeatedly. Because prevalence of chronic bacterial prostatitis is low in the population of men with symptoms associated with chronic prostatitis, the four-specimen test probably should be reserved for men who repeatedly demonstrate increased numbers of leukocytes in expressed prostatic secretions. In men with documented chronic bacterial prostatitis, the ejaculate should also be analyzed to determine the scope of involvement of the male accessory glands. Long-term treatment with culture-specific antibiotics, typically trimethoprim/sulfamethoxazole or the fluoroquinolones, can produce cure rates of 30% to 70%. In one study, the cure rate was more than 90% following short-term intramuscular kanamycin therapy (1000 mg given intramuscularly twice daily for days), followed by 500 mg twice daily for an additional

11 days, and 5 months of either trimethroprim 160 mg/sulfamethoxazole 800 mg orally twice daily, trimethoprim alone 100 mg orally three times daily, or ciprofloxacin 500 mg orally twice daily for patients refractory to short-term kanamycin therapy. If this regimen does not achieve a cure (defined as sterile urine and prostatic secretion culture for at least 12 months after completion of treatment), long-term suppressant antimicrobial therapy must be used to prevent recurrent symptomatic urinary tract infection. Popular suppressive regimens include trimethoprim/sulfamethoxazole 80/400 one tablet orally daily or nitrofurantoin 100 mg orally once or twice daily.

When inflammation as defined by examination of prostatic secretions is documented but the four-specimen test fails to yield an offending organism, a diagnosis of nonbacterial prostatitis is made. It is presumed that nonbacterial prostatitis is caused by an infectious agent that has yet to be identified or by a noninfectious form of prostatic inflammation. A role for *Chlamydia trachomatis* and *Ureaplasma urealyticum* has been proposed for this entity but has not been established. Therefore, routine culture for these agents is recommended only when urethritis is suggested by the patient's history. Some investigators feel that if there is a strong suspicion of ureaplasma or chlamydial infection, a course of minocycline 100 mg orally twice daily or erythromycin 500 mg orally four times daily should be initiated for 14 days. In the absence of a documented source of infection, supportive therapy can be initiated. Such therapy includes increased fluid intake; sitz baths; eliminating such irritating substances from the diet as alcoholic beverages and spicy foods; ejaculation once or twice weekly; analgesics and antiinflammatory agents; and supportive psychotherapy, which is important in the management of any chronic condition. All of these therapies are recommended and yield variable results. Clinical trials using transurethral microwave-induced thermotherapy as palliative therapy have shown promising results.

Granulomatous prostatitis is a rare variant of chronic prostatitis characterized by an extremely indurated texture on digital rectal examination that mimics prostate cancer. While this entity may be idiopathic, it is often associated with previous urinary tract infection; transurethral prostatectomy; needle biopsy of the prostate; or, more recently, with the use of intravesical BCG therapy for bladder cancer. While comprising only 1% of all benign inflammatory conditions of the prostate, a TRUS and biopsy of the prostate are mandatory to rule out prostate cancer.

Finally, prostatodynia remains a diagnosis of exclusion with an uncertain etiology and no proven uniform treatment strategies. Certainly, these patients need to be referred initially to a urologist, in order to confirm the diagnosis and rule out other causes of irritative symptoms of the lower urinary tract, including carcinoma *in situ* of the bladder and interstitial cystitis. However, for carefully selected patients, clinical trials using α-blockers alone or in combination with diazepam are currently underway and have shown some promise. Because antibiotic therapy is ineffective, it should be avoided so that the patient will not fixate on nonexistent somatic causes for the problem.

Suggested Reading

Barry MM and others: The American Urological Association Symptom Index for benign prostatic hyperplasia, *J Urol* 148:1549, 1992.

Benign Prostatic Hyperplasia Guideline Panel: Benign Prostatic Hyperplasia: Diagnosis and Treatment, Clinical practice guideline Number 8, Rockville, MD, U.S. Department of Health and Human Services, 1994.

Bostwick DG (ed): Pathology of the prostate. *Contemporary Issues in Surgical Pathology,* ed 15, New York, Churchill Livingstone, 1990.

Chisholm GD (ed): *Handbook on Benign Prostatic Hyperplasia,* ed 1. New York, Raven Press, 1994.

Chute CG and others: The prevalence of prostatism: a population-based survey of urinary symptoms, *J Urol* 150:85–89, 1993.

Gormley GJ and others: The effect of finasteride in men with benign prostatic hyperplasia: the Finasteride Study Group, *New Engl J Med* 327(17):1234–1236, 1992.

Guess H: Benign prostatic hyperplasia: antecedents and natural history, *Epidemiol Rev* 14:131–153, 1992.

Lepor H, Lawson K (eds): Prostate Diseases, ed 1, Philadelphia, WB Saunders, 1993.

Lepor H and others: A randomized, placebo-controlled multicenter study of the efficacy and safety of terazosin in the treatment of benign prostatic hyperplasia, *J Urol* 148: 1467–1474, 1992.

Weidner W, Madsen PO, Schiefer HG (eds): *Prostatitis: Etiopathology, Diagnosis and Therapy,* ed 1, New York, Springer-Verlag, 1994.

7

Prostate Cancer

Prostate cancer is the most common nondermatologic malignancy in men in the United States and is second only to lung cancer as a cause of death due to cancer. The American Cancer Society estimates that in 1995 there will be 244,000 new cases of prostate cancer diagnosed and over 40,000 deaths directly attributable to prostate cancer. Moreover, on the basis of autopsy studies, it is estimated that approximately 11 million men in the United States older than 45 years of age harbor histologic (clinically silent) prostate cancer. Black men represent a particularly high risk group. The incidence of prostate cancer in American Blacks is 50% higher than in Caucasians. Further, stage-for-stage, five-year survival rates for Blacks are consistently lower than those observed in Caucasian controls.

A second high-risk group is men with a strong family history of prostate cancer. Hereditary prostate cancer is characterized by early age at onset and autosomal dominant inheritance. The gene (or genes) responsible for hereditary prostate cancer have yet to be identified, although this is an active area of research. Two observations suggest that the significant health problem posed by prostate cancer will continue to expand in scope. The frequency of prostate cancer increases with age more than in any other type of cancer. The percentage of men older than 65 years of age in the United States is expected to increase by 64% by the year 2000; therefore, the potential exists for prostate cancer to more seriously impact the male population of the United States in the near future.

PATHOLOGY AND ETIOLOGY

More than 95% of all types of prostate cancer is adenocarcinoma originating in the epithelium that lines the prostatic acinar duct. The other 5% comprises transitional cell carcinomas, squamous cell carcinomas, and carcinosarcomas.

The crucial role of androgens in the development of prostate cancer has been demonstrated in studies that proved that eunuchs do not contract prostate cancer. However, studies that attempt to demonstrate a causal relationship between circulating androgen levels and prostate carcinogenesis have not been convincing. The presence of a genetic component in prostate carcinogenesis is supported by the observation that a hereditary form of the disease affects approximately 10% of men with prostate cancer. Men with first-degree relatives affected by prostate cancer are twice as likely to develop prostate cancer as men without affected first-degree relatives. The clinical and pathologic features of hereditary prostate cancer do not differ significantly from those of the sporadic form of the disease. Linkage studies have been initiated in an attempt to identify the hereditary prostate cancer gene, but candidate loci have yet to be identified.

In many solid tumors, such as colon cancer, benign growths are precursors of malignant tumors. Interestingly, this does not appear to be the case in prostate cancer. No studies have identified a direct relationship between benign prostatic hyperplasia and the development of adenocarcinoma of the prostate. However, prostatic intraepithelial neoplasia, another nonmalignant lesion of the prostate, is closely associated with development of prostate cancer. Patients with prostatic intraepithelial neoplasia diagnosed by needle biopsy of the prostate should be followed very closely, and a second biopsy should be performed to rule out the presence of prostate cancer.

Japanese men and Blacks living in Africa have a relatively low incidence of prostate cancer. Population-based studies show that when Japanese men and African Blacks migrate to the United States, risk for the development of prostate cancer increases. This observation suggests that environmental factors play a significant role in prostate carcinogenesis (Table 7–1). Although case control studies have implicated dietary fat as a risk factor for prostate cancer, cohort studies do not consistently confirm this association. Other environmental factors have been suggested, including low exposure to ultraviolet light, which has been reported to influence prostate carcinogenesis by its effect on vitamin D levels, exposure to heavy metals or infectious agents, and smoking. To date, no consistent data support any single environmental agent as an etiologic factor in prostate carcinogenesis.

Recently, genetic alterations have emerged as important determinants of malignant transformation. The molecular genetic alterations that result in expression of a malignant phenotype are best understood for colon cancer, which serves as the paradigm for molecular carcinogenesis. However, very few consistent genetic alterations have been identified in primary human prostate cancers. Moreover, genes that have been found to play an important role in many other tumors,

TABLE 7–1.

Risk Factors for Prostate Cancer

Established	Suspected
Age	Dietary fat content
Race (Black)	Cadmium exposure
Family history	Vasectomy
	Benign prostatic hyperplasia
	Decreased ultraviolet light exposure

including p53, retinoblastoma gene, and ras oncogene, are not believed to play a significant role in prostate carcinogenesis. Thus, while the etiology of many tumors has been elucidated, the cause of prostate cancer remains a mystery.

CLINICAL PRESENTATION

In the early stages, prostate cancer is asymptomatic. Early cases are often diagnosed on digital rectal examination during a routine physical examination or during examination for some other illness. The recent discovery of prostate-specific antigen (PSA) has profoundly affected the clinical presentation of prostate cancer. Since 1988, this antigen has been widely available as a serum marker for prostate cancer. PSA is a serine protease produced only by prostatic epithelium. Although produced by both normal and malignant cells, the contribution to serum levels differs greatly for these two cell populations. The contribution to serum PSA by benign prostatic hyperplastic tissue is 0.3 ng/ml for each cc of tissue present, while the contribution from prostate cancer tissue is 3.5 ng/ml for each cc of tissue present.

Prostate-specific antigen has been shown to have significant prognostic value. Elevations in this antigen are positively correlated with increasing clinical stage, Gleason grade, and pathologic stage. Furthermore, men with preoperative serum PSA levels of 10 ng/ml or higher have a far greater risk of developing a postoperative recurrence. Elevations of PSA should be interpreted with some degree of caution, however, because such benign conditions as prostatitis and benign prostatic hyperplasia can cause significant increases in the level of PSA in serum. PSA is nevertheless an invaluable asset in the clinical evaluation of men with benign or malignant neoplasms of the prostate.

The normal range for PSA is 0 to 4 ng/ml (Hybertech assay). Values greater than 10 ng/ml strongly suggest but are not diagnostic of prostate cancer. Values between 4 and 10 ng/ml represent a clinical dilemma because the specificity of PSA is poor in this range. A number of assay modifications have been proposed in an attempt to improve the predictive value of PSA in the 4 to 10 ng/ml range. Benson and coworkers used ultrasonography to measure prostate volume and then calculated the amount of PSA per unit volume of tissue to develop a measurement they have termed *PSA density* or PSAD. A PSAD of 0.150 or greater with a PSA between 4 and 10 ng/ml suggests that a needle biopsy of the prostate is indicated regardless of the findings of the digital rectal examination. Such biopsies should be performed with transrectal ultrasonographic guidance. Working with the Baltimore Longitudinal Study of Aging, Carter and associates measured the change in serial PSA on historical samples from men with known outcomes. This has been termed *PSA velocity* (PSAV) or rate of change. They determined that a PSA velocity of 0.75 ng/ml/yr had a high correlation with the presence of clinically significant prostate cancers. This value has been confirmed by two larger studies. Consequently, there should be a high index of suspicion for the presence of prostate cancer in men with a PSA in the 4 to 10 ng/ml range, serial PSA measurements, and a PSAV of 0.75 ng/ml/yr. Oesterling has defined age-associated reference ranges for PSA values. Based on the observation that PSA increases with age, that lower values of PSA might indicate the presence of a cancer that does not need to be treated in an older individual, and allowing for the possibility that lower values of PSA might be ominous in younger individuals, Oesterling has recommended the following normal values for PSA: 0 to 2.5 ng/ml for men aged 40 through 49, 0 to 3.5 ng/ml for men aged 50 through 59, 0 to 4.5 ng/ml for men aged 60 through 69, and 0 to 6.5 ng/ml for men aged 70 and older.

Each of these recommendations has inherent disadvantages and no consensus has been reached in the urologic community concerning their acceptance. PSAD is hampered by the inability of current radiologic techniques to precisely measure prostatic volume and by the wide variance in prostatic epithelial stromal ratios. The age-specific reference ranges were determined in a single community and attempts to generalize these data to other populations have yielded inconsistent results. The usefulness of PSA velocity has been limited because the optimal interval for PSA measurement has not been determined.

Most PSA molecules in the bloodstream are bound to α_1-antichymotrypsin. Recently, it has been shown that significantly less PSA derived from BPH than from prostate cancer circulates in the bound form. As a result, the ratio of bound PSA to free PSA provides a means of differentiating prostate cancer from benign prostatic hyperplasia. At this time, the ratio of bound PSA to free PSA appears to be the best aid to clinical judgment in evaluating men with a normal digital rectal examination and a PSA between 4 and 10.

PSA is believed to be the most valid and sensitive serum marker available for any solid tumor, and its most valuable use is as a posttherapy marker. After definitive treatment for organ-confined prostate cancer, the serum PSA should fall to an undetectable level. A subsequent PSA elevation is pathognomonic for tumor recurrence, although such elevation commonly precedes clinical evidence of local recurrence or distant metastasis. Similarly, patients treated with hormonal ablation for advanced prostate cancer frequently respond with marked reductions in PSA, although the levels remain detectable. Failure of hormone therapy to control the disease generally is first indicated by a rising PSA level. Consequently, measuring serial serum PSA levels is the most sensitive way to monitor the progress of patients treated for both localized and advanced prostate cancer.

Historically, prostatic acid phosphatase has been used as a marker of advanced prostate cancer. The increased sensitivity of PSA and the extreme specificity of PSA elevations in patients with a diagnosis of prostate cancer have resulted in a markedly decreased need for prostatic acid phosphatase measurements.

Despite technologic advances in radiologic techniques to image the prostate and metastatic prostate cancer, approximately 35% of men believed to have clinically localized prostate cancer do not have organ-confined disease at the time of radical prostatectomy. The realization that PSA can help detect prostate cancer at an earlier stage than was previously possible has led to its use as a screening test for prostate cancer. In five large studies of PSA as a screening test, the sensitivity ranged from 46% to 89.5%, and the specificity ranged from 59% to 91.2%. The low sensitivity in these studies precludes the use of PSA alone as a screening test for prostate cancer. However, when combined with a

PROSTATE CANCER SCREENING ALGORITHM

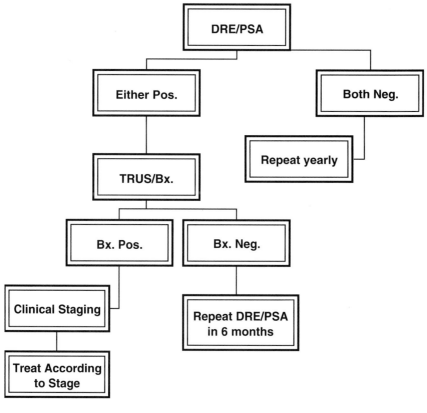

FIG. 7–1.

Algorithm for prostate cancer screening. DRE = digital rectal examination, PSA = prostate-specific antigen, TRUS = transrectal ultrasound, Bx = biopsy.

digital rectal examination, PSA can lead to significantly greater sensitivity and specificity in the early detection of prostate cancer. This has prompted the development of algorithms using PSA, digital rectal examination, and TRUS for early diagnosis of prostate cancer (Fig. 7–1).

Screening for prostate cancer is a controversial issue. To date, no study has been able to document a survival benefit in men diagnosed via screening programs. Prostate cancer is a slow-growing tumor, and screening programs are relatively new. As a result, there is insufficient follow-up time to critically analyze the impact of prostate cancer screening on patient survival.

Despite growing efforts to identify men with early-stage prostate cancer, 20% to 25% continue to present with advanced-stage disease. At the time of diagnosis, these men may have hematuria, lower urinary tract obstruction, or pain from metastasis of the cancer to bone. The axial skeleton, particularly the pelvis and lumbar spine, is most susceptible to metastatic prostate cancer. Another site of metastasis includes the seminal vesicles, by local extension, and spread to the obturator and external iliac nodes can occur via the lymphatic system. Visceral metastasis is less common but can occur in the liver, lungs, adrenal glands, and brain.

DIAGNOSIS AND STAGING

The histologic diagnosis of prostate cancer is made by transrectal biopsy of the prostate. This can be performed on an outpatient basis using local anesthesia (lidocaine gel), with oral antibiotic prophylaxis (fluroquinolone) initiated the night before the procedure. Biopsies in the setting of elevated PSA without obvious findings on digital rectal examination should be performed with transrectal ultrasonographic guidance when possible. Ultrasonography occasionally reveals prostate cancer as a hypoechoic lesion; however, the presence of a hypoechoic lesion is not pathognomonic for prostate cancer, nor does its absence rule out the disease. For a prostatic nodule or induration that is readily palpable, digitally guided biopsies are adequate. Once the presence of prostate cancer is confirmed on a biopsy specimen, the tumor is assigned a grade. The most common grading system in use today is the Gleason system. This system is based on the glandular architecture of the two most commonly seen patterns in the tumor. Both patterns are given a Gleason grade from 1 to 5, with 1 being the most differentiated. The sum of the two grades is the Gleason score. The Gleason score can thus range from 2 to 10 (Fig. 7–2). The Gleason score remains one of the most accurate prognostic indicators for prostate cancer survival.

Clinical staging is used to determine the initial mode of therapy. Radiologic modalities to evaluate pelvic lymph nodes are of little benefit in the staging of prostate cancer. Clinical staging of prostate cancer can be accomplished with

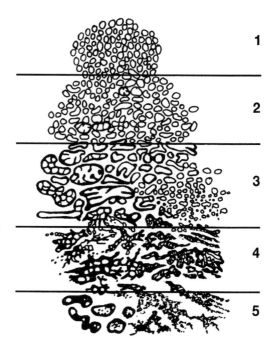

FIG. 7–2.

Gleason system for grading prostate cancer. From Gleason DF: Histologic grading and clinical staging of carcinoma of the prostate, in Tannenbaum M (ed): *Urologic Pathology: The Prostate,* Philadelphia, Lea & Febiger, 1977, pp 171–197.

digital rectal examination, radionucleide bone scan, PSA, and findings on transurethral prostatectomy when appropriate. The TNM staging system for prostate cancer is the currently accepted standard (Fig. 7–3). Organ-confined tumors are designated either T1 or T2. The ability to palpate the tumor on digital rectal examination is the feature that separates these groups. T1 tumors are nonpalpable tumors diagnosed by transurethral resection of the prostate (TURP) or biopsy performed for an elevated PSA only (T1c). T1 tumors detected during TURP are subdivided into two groups on the basis of the percentage of resected cancerous tissue: T1a 5% or less and T1b more than 5%. This distinction has prognostic significance. Of men with untreated T1a disease, 16% will develop metastatic disease within 10 years, while 35% of men with T1b disease will have metastatic disease after five years, and 20% will die of prostate cancer in 5 to 10 years. Palpable T2 tumors are further stratified with respect to the size of the nodule. In T2a disease, the tumor involves less than one half of a lobe; in T2b disease, the tumor involves more than one half of one lobe; and in T2c disease, the tumor involves both lobes. The T3 designation applies to local metastasis outside the prostate. T3a tumors have unilateral extracapsular extension, T3b tumors have bilateral extracapsular extension, and the T3c designation indicates seminal vesicle involvement. T4 tumors have greater degrees of local extension with involvement of contiguous organs (Fig. 7–3).

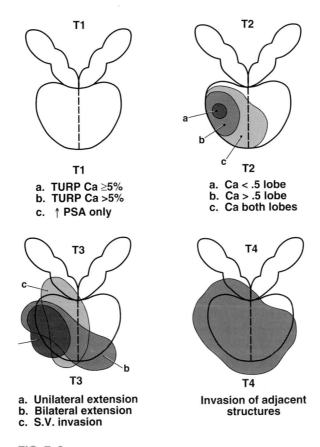

T1

a. TURP Ca ≥5%
b. TURP Ca >5%
c. ↑ PSA only

T2

a. Ca < .5 lobe
b. Ca > .5 lobe
c. Ca both lobes

T3

a. Unilateral extension
b. Bilateral extension
c. S.V. invasion

T4

Invasion of adjacent
structures

FIG. 7–3.

The TNM staging system for prostate cancer. Ca = cancer,
PSA = prostate-specific antigen, SV = seminal vesicle, TURP =
transurethral resection of the prostate.

TREATMENT

Clinically Localized Disease

The treatment of prostate cancer is dictated by the clinical stage of the disease at
the time of diagnosis as well as the patient's age and general health. Patients in
good general health who have T1 or T2 disease and are younger than 70 years of
age are good candidates for curative treatment in the form of radiation therapy or
radical prostatectomy. One can expect a five-year recurrence rate of approximately
20% in patients undergoing radical prostatectomy for disease staged at T2 or less.

A similarly staged group of patients treated with radiation therapy will have a 45% local recurrence rate. Moreover, 30% to 65% of patients treated with radiation therapy will have positive prostate needle biopsies 18 months after treatment. Mortality associated with the treatments are similar—fewer than 1% of patients will die as a result of either therapy. The principal morbidities associated with treatment of localized prostate cancer are impotence and urinary incontinence. In patients 70 years of age or younger, 30% to 60% will be left impotent regardless of the mode of therapy. The incontinence rate after radiation therapy is approximately 2%; the rate associated with radical prostatectomy ranges from 2% to 10%.

Recent surgical advances allow radical prostatectomy to be performed in a bloodless field that allows a full view of the neurovascular bundles that supply innervation to the penis. *Anatomic radical prostatectomy* has substantially reduced the morbidity associated with radical prostatectomy. The decreased morbidity seen with the anatomic approach to radical prostatectomy, coupled with the greater recurrence rate seen with radiation therapy, has resulted in the emergence of radical prostatectomy as the overwhelmingly preferred treatment for men with localized prostate cancer and who are expected to live at least 10 more years.

With the widespread availability of PSA evaluation, prostate cancer is now diagnosed earlier and with greater frequency. Autopsy studies consistently show that one-third of men older than 50 years of age harbor histologically identifiable prostate cancer cells. This percentage increases to 60% of men 90 years of age or older. These types of studies document the presence of a large population of asymptomatic men with prostate cancer who never suffer any adverse effects from the disease. This information has prompted some investigators to suggest that cancers diagnosed by PSA alone (T1C) may be clinically insignificant and not require treatment. In addition, recent studies imply that watchful waiting is adequate for men with localized prostate cancer.

Although provocative, these studies have been less than optimal for the following reasons: 1) hormone therapy has not been used routinely among participants, 2) the mean age of patients enrolled in these studies has generally been 70 years or older, 3) some patients would not have been treated aggressively under standard guidelines, and 4) the studies were biased toward patients with low-grade disease. Recently, Epstein and others reviewed the pathologic findings of 157 consecutive patients with clinical stage T1C disease. These authors found that 84% of tumors were significant and that definitive treatment was justified in a majority of cases. The parameters suggesting that treatment may not be indicated include a PSAD of less than 0.1 ng/ml, Gleason score of 6 or less, and tumor smaller than 3 millimeters on needle biopsy. Patients with tumors not meeting these criteria should be treated with either radical prostatectomy or radiation therapy.

At the present time, the biologic potential of a given tumor cannot be reliably predicted. Consequently, all men with localized prostate cancer who are expected to live at least 10 more years should be offered curative therapy for their disease. Moreover, no evidence exists to suggest that young, healthy patients do not benefit from aggressive treatment of prostate cancer.

Clinically Advanced Disease

Stage T3 tumors extend through the prostate capsule, and 50% to 80% of patients will have disease that metastasizes to the lymph nodes. Because there is no proven adjuvant therapy for prostate cancer, these patients do not benefit from radical prostatectomy. In order to achieve local control of the disease, external beam radiation therapy may be offered.

At present, patients with metastatic disease cannot be cured, and treatment efforts for this group are palliative. Hormone therapy via castration, the use of a gonadotropin-releasing hormone agonist, or administration of estrogen therapy should be implemented with the development of symptoms of metastatic disease. The timing of hormone therapy does not appear to affect survival. Some investigators believe that early initiation of hormone therapy, at the expense of loss of libido and sexual function, can result in increased survival. Others believe that little or no benefit is derived from early hormonal therapy and prefer to withhold such treatment until patients become symptomatic.

Endeavors to develop effective chemotherapeutic regimens for prostate cancer have been disappointing. At this time, no effective chemotherapeutic regimens are in routine use in the treatment of prostate cancer. Two regimens that hold some promise include combination therapy with estramustine phosphate and VP16, two agents that act at the level of the nuclear matrix, and single-agent therapy with suramin, a growth-factor inhibitor.

Complications of advanced prostate cancer that may require surgical intervention include urethral obstruction and spinal cord compression caused by metastasis to lower vertebrae. Urethral obstruction can be treated with transurethral resection of the prostate. Use of lasers or, more recently, the Vaportrode® electrocoagulation instrument allows performance of this procedure with considerably less bleeding than was previously possible. Neurologic symptoms in the lower extremities may signal spinal cord compression in patients with metastatic prostate cancer. If hormone therapy has not been instituted, initial therapy should be orchiectomy; if hormone therapy has been instituted and the patient has a castrate testosterone level, steroids should be administered and neurosurgical consultation obtained to assess the need for laminectomy to surgically decompress the lesion.

Conclusion

Prostate cancer is currently the most common nondermatologic cancer in men. With the increasing age of the U.S. population, prostate cancer looms as one of the major health problems of the 1990s. Recent advances, such as PSA testing and nerve-sparing (anatomic) radical prostatectomy, have considerably improved the care of patients with localized prostate cancer. Unfortunately, treatments for advanced prostate cancer are largely ineffective. The role of the primary-care physician in the treatment of this disorder is to maintain a high index of suspicion in men older than 50 years of age and perform a yearly PSA evaluation and digital rectal evaluation in this group. Men in a high-risk group (i.e., Blacks or men with a family history of prostate cancer) should be evaluated beginning at 40 years of age. These recommendations are supported by the American Cancer Society and the American Urological Association. Men found to have abnormalities on the digital rectal examination or a PSA level of 4.0 ng/ml or greater should be referred to a urologist for further evaluation.

Suggested Reading

Brawer MK: How to use prostate-specific antigen in the early detection or screening for prostatic carcinoma, *CA Cancer J Clin* 45:148–64, 1995.

Carter HB, Coffey DS: The prostate: an increasing medical problem, *Prostate* 16:39–48, 1990.

Catalona WJ and others: Detection of organ-confined prostate cancer is increased through prostate-specific antigen-based screening, *JAMA* 270(8):948–954, 1993.

Catalona WJ: Management of cancer of the prostate, *N Engl J Med* 331(15):996–1004, 1994.

Gann PH, Hennekens CH, Stampfer MJ: A prospective evaluation of plasma prostate-specific antigen for detection of prostatic cancer, *JAMA* 273(4):289–294, 1995.

Narayan, Perinchery: Neoplasms of the prostate gland, in Tanagho EA, McAninch JW (eds): *Smith's General Urology,* Norwalk, CN, Appleton & Lange, 1992, pp 378–412.

The U.S. Preventive Services Task Force: Screening for prostate cancer: commentary on the recommendations of the canadian task force on the periodic health examination. *Am J Prev Med* 10(4):187–192, 1994.

8

Erectile Dysfunction: Diagnosis and Treatment

Impotence is a problem that affects approximately 20 million Americans. Indeed, most men suffer from some degree of impotence at one time or another. The condition can be defined as the inability to attain or maintain an erection adequate for vaginal penetration and sexual intercourse. It is now more appropriately termed *erectile dysfunction*. Erectile dysfunction is different from ejaculatory dysfunction, although the two may be indirectly related. Libido, or the desire to have sex, is another aspect of sexual dysfunction but is not directly related to erectile dysfunction.

Impotence has been ignored and repressed by the medical and the lay communities until relatively recently. In the past, most patients suffering from erectile dysfunction were told that the condition was probably due to psychogenic causes and might improve with counseling or that it was caused by the aging process and was therefore inevitable. As a result of research performed within the past 15 years, we now have a better understanding of the physiology of the erectile process. Through more sophisticated monitoring and physiologic testing, it has become apparent that, in a significant number of patients, problems that were thought to be psychogenic in nature are in fact caused by organic dysfunction.

ERECTILE PHYSIOLOGY

Physiologic studies on a variety of animals, including dogs and monkeys, have clearly demonstrated that erection is caused by arterial dilatation, venous constriction, and relaxation of the corpora cavernosa sinusoids. Histologic studies reveal that the arteries, veins, and corpora cavernosa sinusoids are made of smooth muscles, and these muscles are the prime targets of the neurotransmitters that are released when erection-controlling nerves are stimulated. Acetylcholine, vasoactive intestinal polypeptide, and nitric oxide are believed to be the principal postganglionic neurotransmitters that cause relaxation in the smooth muscles. Upon appropriate sexual stimulation, the neurotransmitters at the level of the penis cause the relaxation of the corporeal smooth muscles, dilatation of the sinusoids and corporeal arteries, and massive increase in blood flow into the sinusoids. The sinusoids then fill with blood, become distended, and compress the draining venules between the external sinusoids and the tunica albuginea, thereby trapping the blood (Fig. 8–1). The intracorporeal pressure rises higher than 100 mm Hg with contraction of the ischiocavernosus muscles.

An erection depends on normal penile anatomy (e.g., elasticity of the tunica albuginea), vasculature, and nerve supply. Detumescence usually occurs after increased sympathetic discharge with associated contraction of the corporeal arteries, decreased blood flow into the penis, and decompression of the draining veins. Diseases that compromise the tunica and adjacent tissues, such as Peyronie's disease, are associated with a loss of venous-occlusive ability and resul-

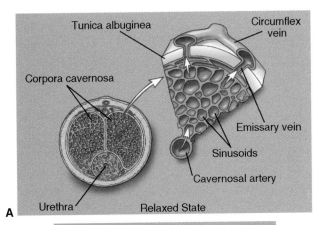

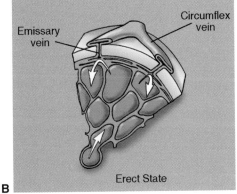

FIG. 8–1

A, Cross section of penis with a triangular segment of corpora cavernosa. In the flaccid state, blood flows from the central corporal artery through the sinusoids and empties through the open emissary veins. Sinusoids are contracted in the flaccid state. **B,** In the erect state, sinusoid smooth muscles are relaxed and blood flows into the sinusoids, but because of distention of the sinusoids against the draining veins, blood becomes trapped in the corporal space.

tant corporeal leakage. Similarly, replacement of the smooth muscles of the sinusoids by collagen results in lack of relaxation and associated erectile dysfunction (Fig. 8–2). Compromised arterial inflow as a result of atherosclerosis or vascular compromise from surgery or pelvic trauma also decreases erectile function. Factors that interfere with nerve conductivity or neurotransmitter release or uptake also affect erections.

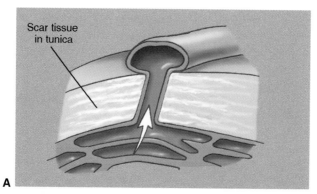

A

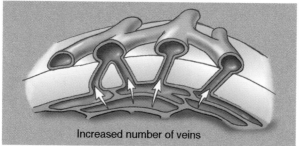

B

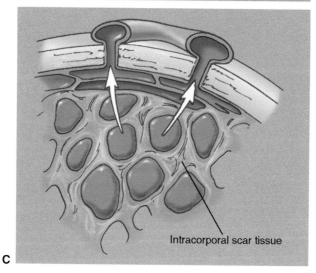

C

FIG. 8–2.

There are three etiologies for corporal venous-occlusive
dysfunction: 1) fibrosis of the tunica albuginea, 2) increased
number of emissary veins, and 3) corporal fibrosis.

EVALUATION OF ERECTILE FUNCTION

The basic elements in the evaluation of erectile dysfunction are a comprehensive history and a thorough physical examination performed in an understanding and empathetic but professional manner. In many instances, the patient will report such nonspecific symptoms as fatigue, voiding dysfunction, and difficulty in sleeping. If the patient's partner is present, her facial expressions may offer the physician a clue to the real problem. Upon questioning, the patient may admit to difficulties achieving or maintaining erections. It is most important to determine the true nature of the problem at this time, that is, to discover whether the patients has lost the desire for sex or is experiencing premature ejaculation, retrograde ejaculation, and delayed orgasms or is unable to achieve or maintain a rigid erection.

After it has been established that erectile dysfunction is the problem, it is important to determine the duration and degree. If the problem has developed gradually, it is likely to be organic in origin, unless some physical event, such as trauma or surgery, transpired immediately prior to onset. It is also important to determine whether erectile dysfunction occurs with all partners or only with the wife, whether the problem is chronic or intermittent, and whether the patient believes that the problem is related to any particular cause. In addition, it is important to determine whether the patient 1) has received medical treatment for the problem, 2) can achieve a sustained erection with masturbation, 3) has rigid nocturnal penile tumescence, or 4) morning "piss hards." If the answers are affirmative, the patient is likely to have psychogenic erectile dysfunction; in some situations, however, when the dorsal nerve of the penis has been traumatized, the patient may achieve erections with central or visual stimulation but be unable to sustain an erection during intercourse.

In other cases, a man may have normal nocturnal penile tumescence and sensual evoked erections but lose rigidity on thrusting movements during intercourse because of the "pelvic steal" syndrome. This occurrence results from partial vascular occlusion above the bifurcation of the iliac arteries, resulting in adequate flow to the pudendal and penile arteries at rest but diversion of some of the penile blood to the gluteal vessels and diminished penile rigidity during thrusting. Asking the patient whether he loses the erection on thrusting or vigorous pelvic movements provides a clue to the situation. Establishing whether the patient has claudication makes it possible to evaluate local blood flow. Penile angulation, nodules, decreased length, and/or pain on erection are suggestive of Peyronie's disease.

Other physical factors that may be disclosed during the history are important chronic medical conditions, such as diabetes mellitus, hypertension, psychologic disorders, endocrine anomalies, peripheral vascular disease, hyperthyroidism or hypothyroidism, neurologic disease, prior surgery, or pelvic trauma. The two

TABLE 8–1.

Drugs Associated
with Erectile Dysfunction

Alcohol	Clofibrate
Antiandrogens	Estrogens
Anticholinergics	Histamine blockers
Antidepressants	Ketoconazole
Antihypertensives	Marijuana
(sympatholytics)	Narcotics
Beta blockers	Psychotropic drugs
Cigarettes	Phenothiazines
and tobacco	Spironolactone
Cocaine	

most common medical causes of erectile dysfunction are diabetes mellitus and peripheral vascular disease. Type I diabetes mellitus accounts for erectile dysfunction in most men who develop the disorder before they reach 45 years of age. Fifty percent of diabetic men older than 50 years of age are organically impotent as a result of either vascular or neurologic problems.

Reviewing the medications, both prescribed and illicit, that the patient is taking may provide pertinent information. Table 8–1 lists the drugs associated with erectile dysfunction. Both antihypertensive and antidepressant agents may contribute to erectile dysfunction. Alcoholism may cause erectile dysfunction by affecting liver function and hormone metabolism as well as by inducing peripheral neuropathies. Smoking and tobacco chewing will cause penile arterial spasm and, on a short-term basis, decrease erectile rigidity. On a long-term basis, these habits expedite the atherosclerotic process. Other contributing factors are marital and/or business stress; extramarital partners; fatigue; and, most commonly, fear of failing to gain an erection. The initial failure may result from any of the factors mentioned and develop into a phobia with resultant subsequent failures. This problem can usually be addressed with counseling and behavior-modification therapy.

The physical examination should be comprehensive and concentrate on the thyroid, penis, testicles, and circulation in the lower extremities. A digital rectal examination of the prostate should also be done. A bulbocavernosus reflex can usually be elicited by simultaneously pinching the glans and sensing the contraction of the anal sphincter. While being stretched, the penis should be examined for plaques and such vesicular lesions as herpes genitalis. Foreskin cracking and frenular irritations, suggestive of chronic balanitis, are usually exacerbated during an erection and can create sufficient discomfort to dissuade continuation of intercourse. The physician should assess the degree to which abdominal obesity may be compromising functional penile length and encourage a weight loss program if appropriate. Testicular size and consistency are other possibly important components to note when evaluating loss of libido and erectile dysfunction.

Having completed the history and physical examination, the physician usually has a fair idea of the etiology of the erectile dysfunction. The next step is to obtain several basic laboratory tests, including urinalysis and evaluation of testosterone, glycohemoglobin, prolactin, cholesterol, and triglyceride levels. Such tests help rule out endocrine or atherosclerotic problems. If the testosterone level is low, the luteinizing hormone and follicle-stimulating hormone levels should be checked to determine whether there is a central (pituitary) or end-organ problem. If the patient does have hypogonadism, a trial of intramuscular Depo®-Testosterone (Upjohn) enanthate injections every three to four weeks would be worthwhile. This regimen should be initiated only if a blood test for prostate-specific antigen is normal.

More refined tests are available to evaluate the neurologic and vascular aspects of the erectile process. These tests are usually within the realm of a urologist and include nocturnal penile tumescence (NPT) testing; penile blood pressure monitoring; biothesiometry to assess vibratory sensation; and duplex Doppler ultrasonographic evaluation of the penile arterial blood flow, both before and after intracorporeal injection of vasodilating agents. Doppler ultrasonography is quite reliable in establishing the status of the arterial inflow in the flaccid and erect state and in determining whether there is evidence of a corporeal leak, which causes inability to trap blood in the corpora. In the event that a leak is suspected, the urologist can perform dynamic infusion cavernosometry and cavernosography (DICC) to establish extent and location.

TREATMENT

Based on the results of the evaluations discussed, the physician can usually determine whether the problem is organic or psychogenic. Psychologic and marital counseling may be effective in patients with psychogenic impotence. However, patients with possible organic etiologies for erectile dysfunction may also have psychogenic impotence, as was the case in a young patient of ours who started to believe that he was developing problems with erectile dysfunction soon after being diagnosed with diabetes mellitus. NPT evaluations were perfectly normal, however, and with reassurance and counseling he regained normal sexual function.

If a patient relates onset of erectile dysfunction to recent initiation of therapy with antihypertensive or antidepressant medications or an histamine blocker, such as Zantac® (Glaxo Pharmaceuticals) or Pepcid® (Merck & Co., Inc.), a change in medications usually solves the problem. At times, a variety of medications must be tried before a reasonable alternative is reached. As mentioned previously, hypogonadism usually can be treated fairly effectively with intramuscular Depo®-Testosterone (Upjohn). If the testosterone level is normal, however, additional supplementation does not improve sexual function. In fact, such supplementation may be deleterious because it inhibits the patient's own production of the hormone. In the presence of significantly elevated cholesterol, administration of cholesterol-lowering medication and initiation of a vigorous exercise and diet program may reverse erectile dysfunction.

A variety of aphrodisiac agents have been on the market for many years. Yohimbine, an indolic alkaloid obtained from the yohimbine tree, has gained partial acceptance by the medical community. This agent is an alpha-2 selective antagonist that enhances norepinephrine release from the nerve terminals by preferential blockade of the presynaptic receptors but minimally interferes with the postsynaptic vascular alpha-1 receptors. A double-blind clinical study of patients with psychogenic impotence showed a 31% response rate with yohimbine versus a 5% response with a placebo. Patients with organic impotence failed to show any statistically significant response.

Agents that increase central concentration of norepinephrine have been found to increase the patient's libido and sexual activity. Such agents include as L-Dopa (catecholamine precursor), deprenyl (a monoamine oxidase-B inhibitor that decreases the breakdown of catecholamines), Sinemet® (DuPont), and amphetamines.

In a study conducted by Heaton and Morales in 1995, apomorphine, a dopamine agonist, was formulated in a proprietary slow-release tablet form and was administered sublingually to a select population of patients with documented psychogenic impotence. Eight of the 12 patients (67%) developed durable erections without side effects with a dose of 3 to 4 milligrams. Further studies are evaluating the potential of this medication.

Trazodone has been used extensively as an antidepressant, and priapism is a recognized potential side effect. Metachlorophenylpiperazine, a metabolite of trazodone, has potent antiserotonin activity and has been shown to induce erections in rats and rhesus monkeys. Clinically, this agent has been reported to cause nocturnal penile tumescence and priapism. In a study by Kurt and associates in 1994, 25 patients with psychogenic impotence were given 50 milligrams of trazodone three times daily for 30 days. Of these patients, 65.2% had a favorable response. In 1992, Bondil suggested combining 25 milligrams of trazodone with 60 milligrams of Moxisylite and administering the combination one hour before sexual activity. He found an improvement in spontaneous sexual activity in 42% of cases. However, these results are from a relatively small population of patients. Multicenter, double-blind studies are planned to confirm the findings.

In the past few years, a variety of topical and intraurethral agents have been evaluated for induction of corporeal vasodilatation. These drugs include topical minoxidil, nitroglycerine paste, and prostaglandin E_1. At present, a multicenter study is being conducted to evaluate miniature suppositories of intraurethral prostaglandin E_1. The preliminary results are promising.

Patients who fail to respond to oral or topical medications may benefit from use of a vacuum erection device. Such devices have gained popularity in the past few years, as the devices have been redesigned to make them easier and safer to use. Long-term results with the vacuum erection device in 217 men with impotence attributed to a wide variety of causes showed satisfaction rates of 84% according to Cookson and Nadig. These devices are not recommended for patients taking anticoagulants or aspirin. A significant number of men, however, find the device inconvenient and painful. Many patients complain of the loss of spontaneity and tend to lose interest in the device. These patients can then be offered either topical or intracorporeal vasodilators that will tend to short-circuit the nervous control of the erectile process and induce erections. These aids, along with psychologic counseling, help the patient overcome the fear of failure, the most common cause of psychogenic erectile dysfunction.

Intracorporeal injections of vasodilators, such as papaverine hydrochloride, phentolamine, and prostaglandin E_1 (individually or in combination) have become very important weapons in the urologist's treatment of erectile dysfunction. Although the Food and Drug Administration has not approved these agents for such use, several thousands of patients are benefiting from them. Side effects include priapism, corporeal scarring, local hematoma, and infection. Infection is the most dangerous potential problem but is also the least common. Priapism occurs in as many as 10% of patients, especially those with either neurogenic or psychogenic erectile dysfunction. The prescribing physician should thus be familiar with management of priapism, which may include surgical intervention.

Last resorts for treatment of erectile dysfunction include revascularization and implantation of a penile prosthesis. Revascularization is usually very effective in young patients who sustained perineal trauma with resultant erectile dysfunction. It is not as effective in older patients with nontraumatic erectile dysfunction. Penile prostheses are excellent alternatives and usually provide the patient with a very functional erection for the rest of their lives. The inflatable penile prosthesis provides the most natural-appearing phallus in both the erect and flaccid state. Penile sensation and ejaculation are unaffected by the implants, and children have been fathered by some patients with implants.

CONCLUSION

Erectile dysfunction is a disease that now is amenable to full evaluation and treatment. Patients should no longer feel that they must suffer in silence.

Suggested Reading

Bondil P: The combination of oral trazodone: diagnostic and therapeutic value in impotence. Report of 110 cases, *Progres En Urologie* 2(4):671, 1992.

Cookson MS, Nadig PW: Long-term results with the vacuum constriction device in a clinical practice, *Int J Impotence Res* 4 [Suppl 2]:A105, 1992.

Heaton JP and others: Recovery of erectile function by the oral administration of apomorphine, *Urology* 45:200, 1995.

Kurt U and others: The efficacy of anti-serotoninergic agents in the treatment of erectile dysfunction, *J Urol* 152:407, 1994.

Levine JF and others: Recurrent erections and priapism as a sequela of priapism: pathophysiology and management, *J Urol* 145:764, 1991.

9

Infertility in Men

Evaluation of infertile couples has received increased medical interest because of the growing number of affected couples, a number estimated to be 15% of all couples attempting to have children. In addition, evolving diagnostic techniques have provided important tools for accurate diagnosis and effective treatment of infertile patients. The increasingly widespread use of such assisted reproductive techniques as *in vitro* fertilization, which is now often combined with sperm and egg micromanipulation, has enabled physicians to treat couples whose condition previously seemed hopeless. Studies of the incidence of male-factor infertility in this patient population have demonstrated that, in 30% of cases, the difficulties are solely attributable to one significant male factor. In 20% of couples, male and female factors combined contribute to the problem. In other words, an abnormal male factor contributes to reproductive failure to some extent in 50% of infertile couples.

The role of the primary-care physician in the evaluation of the subfertile male is critical. In many cases, the primary-care practitioner is the first healthcare professional the patient seeks. This physician is thus provided an excellent opportunity to educate the patient about his problem. The role of the primary-care physician in the evaluation of male infertility is threefold: to perform a thorough history and physical examination; to initiate pertinent, cost- and time-effective laboratory tests; and finally, if appropriate, to refer the patient to a specialist.

HISTORY

The role of the history is invaluable and should follow a format that thoroughly evaluates all potential sources of infertility (Table 9–1). Initially, the primary care physician should determine the duration of the infertility and whether other treatment has been attempted. In the past, fertility evaluations were delayed until a couple had been unable to conceive for one year of unprotected intercourse. However, many couples who have chosen to postpone starting a family because of career goals find themselves in a race against the woman's biological clock and will want to avoid a significant delay in their evaluation. In addition, many couples develop significant anxiety after only a few months of failure to conceive. It is now believed that the evaluation of fertility should begin when patients express concern. In addition, both the male and female portions of a fertility work-up should be coordinated in order to determine whether there is a problem and, if so, to identify it in an efficient, cost-effective, and timely fashion.

Other aspects of the initial history should include a notation of conceptions with past or present partners and the age at which they occurred. Difficulty conceiving and previous evaluations or treatments should be noted.

An inquiry regarding sexual habits, which is best made at the initial visit, provides an opportunity for the family practitioner to offer advice. A problem that is frequently identified pertains to the frequency of sexual intercourse. The

TABLE 9–1.
History of the Infertile Male

Male Reproductive History	c. Gonadotropins (Cont.)
Duration of unprotected intercourse	Radiation exposure (work, diagnostic, therapeutic)
Previous conceptions	
Previous infertility evaluations	Chemical exposure (work, therapeutic)
Female Reproductive History	Smoking (marijuana, cigarettes)
Age	Alcohol
Gravida/para	d. Sexual History
Physician's name	Potency/libido
Ovulation with technique to assess	Coital technique
Current status of female infertility evaluation	Timing and frequency of intercourse
	Use of lubricants
Personal History	e. Medication
a. Developmental	Maternal (DES)
Puberty (normal/delayed/ precocious)	Personal use
History of undescended testes	Steroids
History of gynecomastia	**Family History**
b. Surgical	Cystic fibrosis
Pelvic surgery (Y–V plasty to bladder neck, transurethral surgery)	Androgen receptor deficiency
	Hypogonadism
Retroperitoneal surgery	**Endocrine History**
Inguinal surgery (herniorrhapy, orchidopexy)	Headaches, visual disturbances, anosmia
c. Gonadotropins	Excessive growth of hands, feet, jaw
Occupational exposure	Retardation of hair growth (facial, body)
Thermal exposure (saunas, hot tubs, briefs)	Breast changes
	Vasomotor symptoms

optimal timing for intercourse is every 48 hours during the days when ovulation is most likely (usually during the middle of the woman's cycle). The reason for the alternate-day pattern is that sperm ordinarily survive in normal cervical mucus and in cervical crypts for two days, and viable spermatozoa are assured to be present in the 12- to 24-hour period in which the egg is within the fallopian tube and capable of being fertilized.

Coital habits are also an important subject for the primary-care physician to discuss with the patient. Spermatotoxic lubricants (such as K-Y Jelly, Lubifax,

Surgilube, Keri Lotion) and even saliva can impair sperm motility. Other lubricants, such as raw egg white, vegetable oil, safflower oil, peanut oil, and petroleum jelly do not impair *in vitro* sperm motility. Regardless, couples should use lubricant only if necessary and then only in limited amounts.

Knowledge of specific childhood illnesses and disorders can also be critical in the evaluation of the subfertile male. Cryptorchidism, both unilateral and bilateral, frequently is associated with oligospermia. Studies reveal that approximately 30% of men with unilateral cryptorchidism and 50% of men with bilateral cryptorchidism have sperm densities lower than 20 million/ml; however, 81.4% of men with a history of unilateral cryptorchidism are fertile. In contrast, only 50% of men with a history of bilateral cryptorchidism are fertile. The data concerning the timing of the repair of undescended testicles are inconclusive. Orchidopexies done at increasingly earlier stages have not demonstrated a marked improvement in fertility. What is known is that testicles that descend after puberty do not function well, and fertility rates are not improved with postpubertal orchidopexy.

Trauma or a history of unilateral torsion may also adversely affect the testicles. Approximately 30% to 40% of men with a history of testicular torsion have abnormal semen analysis for reasons that remain unclear. A breakdown in the blood-testicle barrier may be the cause, or the testicle susceptible to torsion may have had a preexisting spermatogenic defect (as evidenced by a high incidence of impaired spermatogenesis in a biopsy from a contralateral testis). When trauma or torsion occurs after puberty, there is speculation that resultant infertility may be immunologically mediated.

A history of a delayed or incomplete puberty may be critical in revealing an endocrinologic etiology (such as Klinefelter's syndrome or idiopathic hypogonadism). Similarly, gynecomastia may also suggest an underlying endocrine problem. Medical problems, such as diabetes and multiple sclerosis, should be investigated because of their potential to impair potency and ejaculation.

Prior bladder, pelvic, or retroperitoneal surgery suggests the possibility of ejaculatory dysfunction. In the 1960s, a Y-V plasty of the bladder neck at the time of ureteral surgery was common. Because this bladder surgery ablates the internal urinary sphincter, individuals who undergo the procedure often experience retrograde ejaculation and frequently have an ejaculate volume of less than 1 milliliter. Evaluation of postejaculate urine confirms the diagnosis by revealing large numbers of sperm in a centrifuged specimen. If retrograde ejaculation is detected, the physician can institute a course of alpha-adrenergic medications (such as ephedrine sulfate, 50 mg orally 4 times daily) for 2 weeks to determine whether retrograde ejaculation has been minimized. If is has not, referral to a specialist is warranted.

Men who have been treated for cancer often experience infertility problems. Chemotherapeutic agents (especially alkylating agents, such as cyclophosphamide, mustine, and chlorambucil) are particularly damaging to the germinal epithelium. Also, radiation exposure (which is cumulative) can severely impair fertility. Patients with testicular cancer are particularly affected. Many of these patients choose to have their sperm frozen (sperm banking) prior to initiation of cancer treatment. Patients who have survived the rigors of chemotherapy, radiation therapy, retroperitoneal lymph node dissection (RPLND), or a combination of these treatments often find it necessary to seek help to enhance fertility. Impaired spermatogenesis is a risk for any patient who has been treated with radiation therapy or chemotherapy for testicular cancer or any other type of cancer. Normal spermatogenesis may not return for as long as five years, so aggressive treatment does not need to be considered for that length of time.

Patients who have had a standard RPLND may experience aspermia (lack of a visible ejaculate) or, less frequently, retrograde ejaculation. In the standard RPLND, the sympathetic chain or its long nerves (sacral plexus, hypogastric nerves) may be interrupted in the dissection. New "nerve-sparing" RPLND techniques have significantly decreased this problem—75% of men who have undergone nerve-sparing RPLND have normal antegrade ejaculates. Men with ejaculatory dysfunction after RPLND often benefit from sympathomimetic drugs (such as ephedrine sulfate). If pharmacologic therapy fails, obtaining a semen sample using rectal probe electrostimulation may be attempted for intrauterine insemination or *in vitro* fertilization.

History of a herniorrhaphy suggests the possibility of an iatrogenic vasal injury. In addition, any inflammatory process that involves the lower urinary tract may lead to adverse scarring of the ductal system (e.g., ejaculatory duct stenosis or obstruction) that may affect fertility. It has been reported that 10% of patients who experienced bilateral mumps orchitis after puberty develop severe testicular damage, although mumps orchitis occurring before puberty has no effect. Furthermore, any generalized febrile episode may impair spermatogenesis. Because spermatogenesis requires 74 days from initiation to the appearance of mature spermatozoa, ejaculate may not be affected for approximately three months. Therefore, evaluation of fertility should be delayed for at least three months after a significant febrile event.

Immotile cilia syndrome (nonmotile sperm secondary to an ultrastructural defect in the sperm tail) may be the cause of infertility in men with recurrent respiratory infections. A variant of immotile cilia syndrome, Kartagener's syndrome, is characterized by sinusitis, chronic bronchiectasis, situs inversus, and immotile spermatozoa. Another variant is Young's syndrome (also associated with pulmonary disease) in which the cilia ultrastructure is normal, but the epididymis is blocked because of inspissated material. A great number of men who unknowingly carry a gene for cystic fibrosis have congenital absence of the vasa and seminal vesicles and, therefore, will present with a low ejaculate volume and azoospermia.

History of chemical, pharmacologic, and environmental exposure must be determined. Medications, toxins, and drugs that are associated with infertility in men are listed in Table 9–2. Exposure to lead affects the hypothalamic-pituitary-gonadal axis and results in the suppression of serum

TABLE 9–2.

Medications, Toxins, and Drugs Associated with Male Infertility

Medications	Toxins
Androgenic steroids	Agent Orange
Antihypertensives	Anesthetic gasses
Cancer chemotherapy	Benzene
Histamine blockers	Dibromochloropropane
Ketoconazole	Lead
Nitrofurantoin	Manganese
Spironolactone	**Other Drugs**
Sulfasalazine	Alcohol
Colchicine	Heroin
Allopurinol	Marijuana
Tetracycline	Methadone
Erythromycin	Tobacco
Gentamicin	
Cyclosporine	

testosterone. Dibromochloropropane, once widely used as an agricultural soil fumigant, appears to be a severe testicular toxin. Cigarette smoking may impair fertility by impairing sperm density, motility, and morphology. Marijuana use can lower serum testosterone levels and temporarily reduce sperm density and motility. Alcohol abuse may alter androgen metabolism to produce sexual dysfunction; can reduce serum testosterone; and appears to reduce sperm motility and density and alter normal morphology. Opiate abuse inhibits gonadotropin secretion to decrease serum testosterone. Prenatal exposure to diethylstilbestrol (DES) may increase the incidence of epididymal cysts and slightly increase the frequency of cryptorchidism. Sulfasalazine (frequently used to treat ulcerative colitis) can reduce sperm motility and density, although the condition is reversible. Such drugs as spironolactone, cyproterone, ketoconazole, and cimetidine can inhibit androgen production. Nitrofurantoin (in high doses) depresses spermatogenesis, and tetracycline lowers testosterone levels by as much as 20% during short-term therapy. Antimicrobial agents, such as erythromycin and gentamicin, may impair spermatozoal function and transiently impair fertility. Anabolic steroids, which are often used by athletes, act temporarily and sometimes irreversibly as a "male contraceptive" by depressing gonadotropin secretion.

Environments that increase the overall scrotal temperature should be avoided. The elevated testicular temperature seen in cryptorchidism and in association with scrotal varicoceles may explain the impaired spermatogenesis associated with these disorders. Therefore, it is often recommended that men discontinue the use of tight bikini briefs (in favor of boxers) and avoid the use of saunas and hot tubs to optimize sperm production. However, only the adverse effect of direct heat elevation (e.g., hot tubs) has been scientifically investigated.

PHYSICAL EXAMINATION

The initial physical examination performed by the primary-care practitioner may reveal critical information pertaining to the etiology of a man's infertility. Special care should be taken by the physician to note evidence of hypogonadism (characterized by poor secondary sexual characteristic development, eunuchoidal skeletal proportions, and lack of normal male hair distribution). Evidence of visual field defects, galactorrhea, and headaches may indicate a hypothalamic or pituitary tumor. Also, men with congenital hypogonadism may have associated defects, such as anosmia, color blindness, cerebellar ataxia, harelip, and cleft palate. Gynecomastia may indicate primary testicular failure or a secondary hypothalamic-pituitary-testicular axis abnormality.

Because the seminiferous tubules account for 85% of testicular volume, a careful examination of the testicles may help identify the origin of the infertility, that is, whether it results from testicular or posttesticular (obstructive) causes. The normal adult testicle averages 4.6 centimeters in length, 2.6 centimeters in width, and 18.6 milliliters in volume. These parameters can easily be measured using a ruler, caliper, or orchidometer. If testicular insult has occurred before puberty, the testicles are most likely to be small and firm; damage after puberty usually renders them small and soft.

The prostate should be carefully examined for size (often small in men with androgen deficiency) and consistency (tender and boggy with prostatitis). The penis should be examined for any abnormalities (hypospadias, abnormal curvature, phimosis) that may interfere with the proper deposition of sperm deep within the vagina. The epididymis and vas should be carefully palpated because an irregular epididymis may indicate infection or obstruction, and approximately 2% of infertile men have congenital absence of the vasa and seminal vesicles. Because these men are also at risk for carrying one of more of the genes for cystic fibrosis, they should have a genetic evaluation.

Next, the testicular cords should be carefully palpated for the presence of a varicocele. With the patient standing in a warm examination room, the testicular (spermatic) cord should be palpated between the thumb and index finger while the patient performs the Valsalva maneuver (i.e., takes a deep breath and "bears down"). An increase in the thickness of the cord or the presence of a discrete pulse (the venous reflux) suggests the possibility of a varicocele. In addition, a boggy mass that resembles a bag of worms surrounding the left testicle is characteristic of a large varicocele. When abnormalities are noted on the genital examination, prompt referral to the urologist is indicated for further noninvasive examinations (including ultrasonography) or evaluation for possible surgery. Finally, a full physical examination is performed to rule out chronic or unsuspected systemic diseases that may impair testicular function.

LABORATORY EXAMINATION

The preliminary laboratory examination performed by the primary-care physician should include two properly collected and analyzed semen samples and the evaluation of serum follicle-stimulating hormone (FSH) levels. The importance of proper specimen collection and analysis by a laboratory that has demonstrated quality control in evaluating semen samples and performs at least 20 analyses per week cannot be overemphasized. Analytic techniques can vary by as much as 20%, so the laboratory to which the patient is referred must be chosen carefully. In addition, it must be realized that any laboratory analysis does not predict fertility. Pregnancy is the only irrefutable proof of the sperm's capability to fertilize. If abnormalities are noted in the semen samples, urologic referral is indicated. Elevated FSH likewise suggests intrinsic testicular failure with compensatory increase in FSH production by the pituitary, and the elevated hormone should prompt urologic referral.

Semen Analysis

Semen should be collected for analysis after 48 to 72 hours of abstinence. Ideally, it should be collected at the laboratory by masturbation into a container (furnished by the laboratory) that has been tested to ensure that it will not alter the sperm sample's quality. The specimen should be analyzed within 1 hour and kept at body temperature before analysis in order to ensure accuracy of the evaluation. A minimum of two samples should be obtained. To decrease variability, each sample should be collected after the same period of sexual abstinence (two to three days).

Several characteristics of the semen sample are analyzed, and the parameters for adequately fertile sperm are listed in Table 9–3. First, semen volume is assessed. The normal volume for an ejaculate is between 1.5 to 5.0 milliliters. Fertility appears to be affected only when semen volume drops below 1.5 milliliters, the point at which inadequate buffering of the vaginal acidity occurs. A low-volume sample can be associated with incomplete collection, retrograde

TABLE 9–3.
Semen Analysis: Limits of Adequacy

Ejaculate volume:	1.5 to 5.0 ml
Sperm density:	> 20 million/ml
Percent motility:	> 60%
Forward progression:	> 2 (scale 0 to 4)
Morphology:	> 60% normal forms

ejaculation, ejaculatory duct obstruction, or androgen deficiency. A low volume may result in inadequate sperm-mucus interaction.

Second, the sperm is analyzed for density (concentration). The lower limit of normal believed to be necessary to conceive is 10 to 20×10^6/ml, with a total of 50 million sperm per ejaculate. It cannot be overemphasized that the evaluation may be altered significantly if the two samples are not collected after approximately equal abstinence periods, with each day of abstinence (up to one week) altering the sperm concentration by 10 to 15 million/ml and the total sperm count by 50 to 60 million/ml. In addition, prolonged abstinence may result in lower motility, because the sperm may die with prolonged retention within the male ductal system.

Third, the sample is analyzed for motility. This is the most important measure of semen quality, as evidenced by the fact that patients with hypogonadotropic hypogonadism who have a very low sperm count (<10 million/ml) but highly motile sperm seldom have fertility problems. On the other hand, oligoasthenospermic patients have a low count and poor motility and thus have significant problems with fertility, even when sperm and egg are placed together *in vitro*. Sperm motility is characterized by two equally important measurements: 1) the number of motile sperm as a percentage of the total and 2) the quality of sperm movement or forward progression (how fast and straight the sperm move). The normal motility measured in a semen sample is at least 50% with a forward progression rate of at least 2.0 (the forward progression scale ranges from 0 for no movement to 4.0 for excellent forward progression). An average forward progression is greater than 2.0.

An aliquot of the sample is air dried on a slide and stained for determination of sperm morphology. Normal semen samples contain at least 50% morphologically normal sperm. Increased numbers of abnormally shaped sperm indicate testicular stress (e.g., varicocele, poor sperm production, environmental toxins). The sample should also be analyzed for the presence of leukocytes. Most evidence suggests that pyospermia is detrimental to sperm function and may indicate infection or inflammation. If pyospermia exists, consultation with a urologist is in order.

Further tests of sperm physiology might include the quantification of anti-sperm antibodies, a sperm-cervical mucus interaction test, acrosomal membrane staining, and the sperm penetration test. However, these more complicated assays are best left to a specialist in male reproductive disorders.

Hormone Evaluation (Fig. 9–1)

Primary endocrine defects in infertile men occur at a rate of 3%, and such defects are rare in men whose sperm concentration is greater than 5×10^6/mL. However, when endocrinopathy is suspected, specific hormonal treatment is often successful. Therefore, a hormone evaluation should be performed when the sperm concentration is low or when an endocrinopathy is suspected clinically. This testing can be initiated by the primary-care physician or can be handled entirely by a urologist. Hormone status as it relates to clinical diagnosis is discussed in Table 9–4.

When spermatogenesis is reduced, a generalized decrease in production of inhibin by the Sertoli's cells (support or nurse cells) usually occurs. This decrease in inhibin effectively reduces negative feedback to the pituitary gland and is associated with a reciprocal elevation of FSH. Elevated FSH levels are generally a dependable measure of injury to the germinal epithelium. Marked elevations in serum FSH are usually associated with azoospermia or severe oligospermia and usually indicate a difficult-to-treat germ cell defect (such as primary testicular failure or perhaps hypogonadotropic hypogonadism, the latter of which is suggested clinically by undermasculinization). When correlated with concomitantly decreased levels of serum testosterone and luteinizing hor-

TABLE 9–4.
Hormone Status Correlated to Clinical Diagnosis

Clinical Status	FSH (mIU/ml)	LH (mIU/ml)	Testosterone (ng/100 ml)
Normal men	Normal	Normal	Normal
Germinal aplasia	Elevated	Normal	Normal
Testicular failure	Elevated	Elevated	Normal or decreased
Hypogonadotropic hypogonadism	Decreased	Decreased	Decreased

FSH = follicle-stimulating hormone, LH = luteinizing hormone.

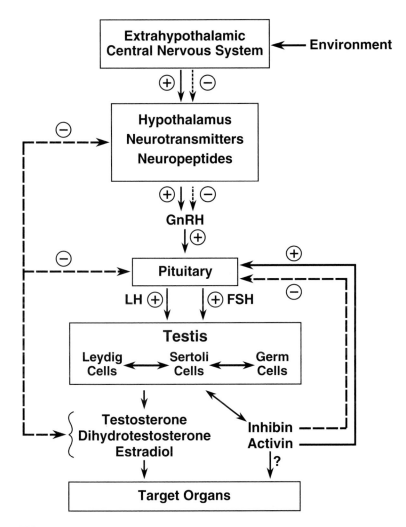

FIG. 9–1.

Diagram of the hypothalamic-pituitary-testicular axis. GnRh = gonadotropin-releasing hormone, LH = luteinizing hormone, FSH = follicle-stimulating hormone. (From Swerdloff RS, Wang C: Physiology of male reproduction: hypothalamic-pituitary function, in Walsh PC and others (eds): *Campbell's Urology,* ed 6, Philadelphia, WB Saunders, 1992, p 177. Reproduced with permission.)

mone, the diagnosis is confirmed and appropriate treatment should be initiated under the direction of a urologist or endocrinologist. A year of hormone therapy may be required before optimal sperm production is reached. Because hyperprolactinemia has also been reported to cause oligospermia, serum prolactin should be measured when a patient has a low serum testosterone level without an associated increase in luteinizing hormone as well as symptoms of decreased libido, decreased ejaculate volume, and galactorrhea.

SPECIALIST REFERRAL

Once a thorough history and physical examination are completed and the appropriate laboratory tests are performed by the primary-care physician, referral to a urologic specialist in the field of male reproductive medicine and surgery can be considered.

CONCLUSION

The importance of the primary-care physician in evaluation of male infertility cannot be overstated. The initial evaluation and laboratory testing process can be critical for an infertile couple, especially for facilitating prompt referral when indicated. Moreover, this is an opportunity to counsel the couple. They should be made aware that the duration of therapy depends on the nature of the problem and that the cost of evaluation and treatment of infertility can be substantial. They should also be informed that the likelihood of conception depends on the cause of the problem. With the proper evaluation and appropriate referral, male-factor problems are being treated at an increasingly successful rate and previously infertile couples are able to enjoy the rewards of parenthood.

Suggested Reading

Gilbert BR, Schlegel PN, Goldstein M: Office evaluation of the subfertile male, *AUA Update Series* 13:69–76, 1994.

Howards SS: Current concepts: treatment of male infertility, *N Engl J Med* 332:312–317, 1995; .

Lipshultz LI (ed): Male infertility, *Urol Clin North Am* 21(3), 1994.

Lipshultz LI, Howards SS, Buch JP: Male infertility, in Gillenwater JY and others (eds): *Adult and Pediatric Urology, ed 2,* St. Louis, Mosby–Year Book, 1991, pp 1425–1478.

McClure RD: Male infertility, in Tanagho EA, McAninch JW (eds): *Smith's General Urology,* Norwalk, Appleton & Lange, 1995, pp 739–770.

Sigman M, Howards SS: Male infertility, in Walsh PC and others (eds): *Campbell's Urology,* Philadelphia, WB Saunders, 1992, pp 659–706.

10

Common Urologic Problems in Children

There are a number of pediatric urologic problems that the family practitioner will encounter when caring for newborn babies and young children. The goal of this chapter is to help the clinician understand, identify, and treat many of these problems. Some children are born with congenital abnormalities (i.e., cryptorchidism, hypospadias, hernias) that will require urologic consultation for possible surgical correction. Of these congenital disorders, cryptorchidism is discussed in detail; other important topics in pediatric urology reviewed in this chapter include hydronephrosis, hydrocele, circumcision, balanoposthitis and balanitis, urinary tract infection, and testicular torsion.

CRYPTORCHIDISM

Cryptorchidism, or undescended testicles, is the most common urologic abnormality found in newborn boys. Approximately 4% of male infants carried to term are born with cryptorchidism; 15% of which are bilateral cases. Within three to six months after birth, testicles descend in 75% of affected babies, probably because of a transient increase in testosterone as mediated by the temporary production of luteinizing hormone (LH) and follicle-stimulating hormone (FSH) at this time. Therefore, at nine months, slightly fewer than 1% of boys have undescended testicles. This figure is constant throughout the remainder of life in untreated boys and men as documented in several studies. After the first nine months of age, spontaneous testicular descent does not occur, and, if described, indicates that the initial diagnosis should be questioned. Recent information suggests an unexplained increase in the incidence of cryptorchidism.

A premature child has an even a greater chance of having the disorder because testicular descent occurs relatively late in gestation. Indeed, the greater the degree of prematurity, the greater the incidence of cryptorchidism. All boys weighing less than 910 grams at birth have undescended testicles, as opposed to only 17% of premature boys weighing more than 2040 grams. Furthermore, in full-term infants, the incidence of cryptorchidism is directly related to weight.

The testicles are formed in the abdomen and descend during the last trimester of pregnancy. There are several theories concerning the etiology of cryptorchidism, none of which has been generally accepted. It is thought that testicular descent depends on several mechanisms, including intraabdominal pressure, the local presence of testosterone, the gubernaculum and its attachment to the scrotum, the appropriate function of the genitofemoral nerve, and the integrity of the epididymis. Experimental evidence supports each of these suggested mediators of testicular descent. Although there is no compelling evidence for any one theory, testicular descent is probably dependent on several interrelated factors.

What is apparent, however, is that normal testicular development is dependent on the testicles being present within the scrotum. The temperature of the scrotum is 2° to 3°C cooler than the abdominal cavity, a difference that is crucial to occurrence of normal spermatogenesis. It has been noted that undescended testicles are often smaller than normally descended partners, and it has been suggested that this is due to the difference in temperature in their location.

The classification of testicular maldescent has been described in several sources and is generally accepted (Fig. 10–1). Retractile testicles, which are a variant of normal, must be distinguished from true cryptorchidism. It has been suggested than the majority of patients referred for evaluation of cryptorchidism actually have retractile rather than undescended testicles. Retractile testicles occasionally reside in the scrotum but are elevated from that position by a hyperactive cremasteric muscle. During physical examination, such testicles can be brought into the scrotum where they will remain for at least several moments before returning to the inguinal region. A significant effort should be made to differentiate these testicles from truly nondescended testicles because treatment is unnecessary for retractile testicles.

The location of undescended testicles can be identified on physical examination. Most undescended testicles (80%) are palpable and located distal to the internal inguinal ring. These can be divided into ectopic and truly undescended testicles; however, the clinical difference between these two is not important. Ectopic testicles have emerged from the external inguinal ring but have deviated from the normal pathway of descent and do not reside in the scrotum. The most common location for these testicles is the superficial inguinal pouch of Denis Browne. Other locations include the perineum, thigh, femoral canal, and prepenile area. In cases of true cryptorchidism, the gonad remains along the normal path of descent but because of shortened or tethered cord structure (testicular vessels or vas deferens), the testicle does not reach the scrotal sac. These testicles are found within the inguinal canal or distal to the external ring but not yet in the scrotum.

Intraabdominal testicles account for approximately 16% of undescended testicles; such testicles reside within the inguinal ring, often just within the abdomen. Others, however, can be found much higher, that is, well within the belly. It seems clear that the higher the testicle, the poorer its ability to reach normal development and subsequent function. The difficulty involved in repairing testicles located high in the abdomen is significant, and the incidence of malignant degeneration is higher. For these reasons, it has been suggested (but is generally not accepted) that if the contralateral testicle is in a normal position, ipsilateral orchiectomy is an appropriate therapy. The remaining 4% of undescended testicles are atrophic or absent. If present, their position can be anywhere along the path of testicular development or descent. As there is no indirect way of determining unilateral absence of a gonad, diagnosis requires either surgical exploration or laparoscopy.

There is no adequate way, short of surgery, to determine the presence or absence of a unilateral cryptorchid testicle in a child. Radiographs and ultrasonography are not reliable, especially in young boys because of the small size of

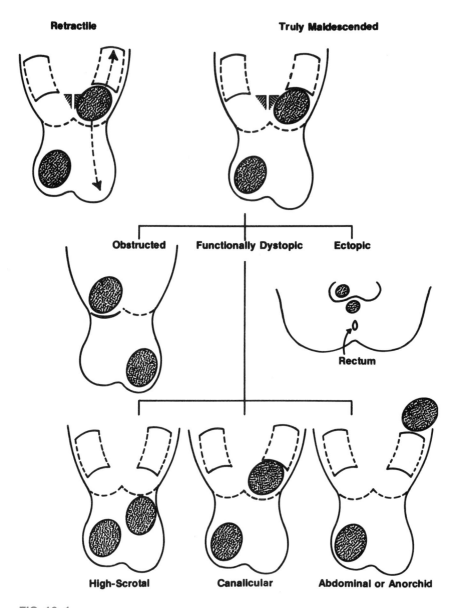

FIG. 10–1.

Types of testicular maldescent. (From Lipshultz LI: Cryptorchidism in the subfertile male, *Fertil Steril* 27:610, 1976. Reproduced with permission of the publisher, the American Society for Reproduction (The American Fertility Society).)

the testicle and the surrounding adipose tissue. In rare cases of nonpalpable bilateral testicles, hormonal evaluation that includes human chorionic gonadotropin (HCG) stimulation (2,000 IU given intramuscularly daily for five days) may preclude the need for surgical exploration. In true bilateral anorchism, elevated levels of both FSH and LH must be present before HCG stimulation and testosterone must not increase after the course of HCG. In those cases, anesthesia can be avoided and the diagnosis of anorchism is made. In cases where testosterone does rise after the course of HCG, either laparoscopy or laparotomy must be performed and the diagnosis of absent testes is made by observation of blind-ending testicular vessels meeting the vas deferens.

Physical Examination

Evaluation of the cryptorchid testicle is generally restricted to physical examination. A complete examination of a newborn should include documentation of the location of the gonads. The examination generally is done with both hands, the dominant one feeling for the testicle while the contralateral hand sweeps in an inferior direction from the anterosuperior iliac spine. It is often helpful if the examiner's hand is wet with soapy water to allow a sliding motion over the inguinal region; at times this enables the physician to identify an otherwise nonpalpable testicle. Once the testicle is identified, an attempt should be made to slide the testicle into the scrotum. If the testicle remains in the scrotum for at least a few seconds, the diagnosis is a retractile testicle. Conversely, if the testicle cannot be brought into the scrotum or if it immediately retracts after being brought into the inguinal region, the diagnosis is an undescended testicle. Attention should be given to making the patient as comfortable as possible before and during the examination. The physician's hands should be warm, and the patient should be examined in different positions, including erect, supine, and squatting.

If the diagnosis of an undescended testicle is made in a newborn, it is best to counsel the family to be patient, because the majority of neonatal cryptorchid testicles spontaneously descend within the first several months of life. If the child is older than six months of age, it is reasonable to discuss treatment with the parents.

An increased incidence of testicular tumors in young men with a history of cryptorchidism has been well documented. It has not been shown that relocating the testicles within the scrotum decreases the incidence of tumors, but a testicle in the normal position can be easily palpated and abnormalities noted so that early treatment can be instituted. There are varying estimates of the risk of testicular cancer associated with an undescended testicle; these estimates range from 4 to 40 times that of the general population's, which is approximately 1:250,000. The most common tumor associated with treated cryptorchidism is a nonseminomatous germ cell tumor, whereas the seminomas are more often seen in intraabdominal testicles. There are no reliable data showing that treatment of a cryptorchid testicle decreases the incidence of malignant degeneration. Indeed, there is an increase in the incidence of cancer in the contralateral normally descended testicle. The reason for this is not understood.

Another concern associated with cryptorchidism is the child's subsequent fertility potential. Several studies have documented decreased sperm counts in men who have a history of unilateral or bilateral cryptorchidism, and the data suggest that an undescended testicle is severely restricted in its ability to produce viable sperm. These studies imply that men with a history of unilateral cryptorchidism have normal paternity rates, although their sperm counts are generally below the accepted normal figure of 20,000,000 per cc. On the other hand, men with a history of bilateral cryptorchidism do have both diminished sperm counts and decreased paternity rates.

Despite several studies documenting changes in sperm parameters in men with a history of cryptorchidism, there is very little information to confirm the beneficial effects of treatment or any specific timing of treatment in boys with undescended testicles. It may be that the paucity of information is related to the relatively short follow-up of boys with very early treatment of cryptorchidism. It is clear that later treatment (i.e., at six years of age or older), probably does not significantly improve paternity or fertility. Only within the past two decades has early intervention been suggested in the treatment of this problem, and paternity data are not yet available from a large cohort of patients who were treated before two years of age. It is hoped that as the boys who received early treatment reach marriageable age, positive effects of treatment, especially in the case of bilateral cryptorchidism, will be identified.

The patient's self-image is another reason to proceed with treatment of cryptorchidism. As the boy becomes an adolescent, he will want to appear like his peers with two descended testicles. In some situations, the asymmetry present with cryptorchidism is so severe that the defect is obvious from a distance. Ridicule in the locker room can be devastating to boys of high-school age, and early correction of the problem is appropriate.

Treatment

Treatment of cryptorchidism may be medical (hormonal) or surgical (Fig. 10–2). Hormone therapy is appropriate initially because testosterone is one of the determinants of testicular descent. In Europe, treatment is often begun shortly after two months of age in an attempt to reconstruct the normal transient increase in hormone levels that occurs at three months of age. Gonadotropin-releasing hormone (GnRH) is given as a nasal spray. The GnRH stimulates the pituitary to produce LH and FSH. LH induces the testicles to manufacture testosterone. The usual dosage of the medication is 200 μg three times a day and the length of treatment is generally four weeks. Success rates of up to 60% have

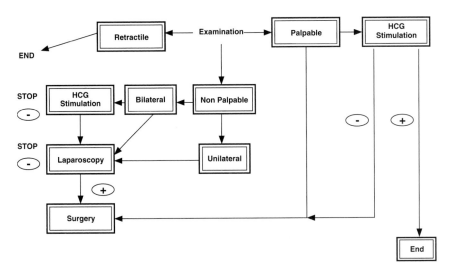

FIG. 10–2.

Algorithm for suggested evaluation and treatment of cryptorchisdism. HCG = human chorionic gonadotropin.

been reported in these young boys. If subsequent treatment with HCG is used, a success rate of 79% has been claimed. These studies, however, have been criticized for lack of controls and inclusion of children with retractile testicles. Other studies, in both the United States and Europe, could not duplicate these excellent results and reported success rates of only 11% to 38%. At this time, GnRH is not approved in the United States for treatment of cryptorchidism.

The hormone HCG is used instead of GnRH in this country in children older than six months of age. The medication must be given intramuscularly and has limited success, especially in infancy. Several dosage schedules are in use. However, the most commonly suggested total dose is between 10,000 and 12,000 IU given intramuscularly over a two- to three-week period. Higher doses over a longer period should be avoided because of the possibility of premature closure of the epiphyseal plates from testosterone. Common side effects stem from the increased testosterone levels and include a slight increase in the size of the penis, early rugation of the scrotum, and the transient appearance of fine pubic hair. Success of treatment depends greatly on the initial location of the gonad. The closer the testicle is to the scrotum, the more likely it is that a favorable response will occur. When the testicle can be manipulated into the scrotum, the success rates have been reported to be as high as 90%, although the possible inclusion of patients with retractile testicles may have distorted this figure. Controversy exists concerning the longevity of initial response to HCG. Studies have described a deterioration of position over time with positive early results giving way to testicular ascent. Therefore, repeated examinations for several months are needed in boys who have undergone treatment with HCG for cryptorchidism.

For boys refractory to hormone therapy or those whose parents refuse such treatment, surgery is the other option. Indeed, parents often elect to proceed directly to surgery once the nature of hormone therapy and its success rate are discussed. In boys with a nonpalpable testicle, there is current enthusiasm for laparoscopy as the initial surgical event. This procedure can be done through a small subumbilical incision and can confirm the absence of a testicle if blind-ending testicular vessels and vas deferens can be found together. In such cases, open surgical exploration can be avoided. If an intraabdominal testicle is noted at laparoscopy, treatment decisions can be instituted to simplify the required surgery. In some centers, the entire orchiopexy is being approached through the laparoscope. However, in most areas, open surgery is undertaken once the nature of the anatomy has been delineated. If the testicle is noted within the abdomen, a higher incision is made, allowing better evaluation and treatment of the gonad. On the other hand, if testicular vessels and vas deferens are seen exiting the abdomen, an inguinal exploration is performed. If vessels and a blind-ending vas deferens are identified in the groin, the operation is terminated and a diagnosis of an atrophic testicle is made. If the testicle is found, orchiopexy is then completed.

Although several procedures have been described for the operative treatment of a palpable undescended testicle, the basic principles of all the procedures are similar. Surgical exploration for the palpable testicle is begun with an inguinal incision. The external oblique fascia is opened, and the inguinal canal is entered. The spermatic cord, including the testicular vessels, vas deferens, and often a hernia sac, is identified. The cord is followed caudally until the gonad is identified and freed of surrounding structures. The hernia is repaired, and the testicle is repositioned in the scrotum. The surgery is done on an outpatient basis, and complications are rare. The most common problems reported are injury to the testicular vessels or vas deferens. Other, less frequent complications include hemorrhage, infection, and the need for orchiectomy. Long-term surgical complications include ascent of the testicle, recurrence of the hernia, or testicular atrophy. The total complication rate should be less than 1%.

More elaborate techniques are used when the testicle is difficult to reposition in the scrotum. Such techniques include dividing the testicular vessels (Fowler-Stephens procedure), staged orchiopexy (in which the gonad is brought as far as possible in the initial operation and a second attempt at positioning in the scrotum is performed in six months), and microvascular repositioning and reanastomosis of the testicular vessels and vas deferens. In addition, recent papers have reported successful endoscopic treatment of intraabdominal testicles.

Given the possible long-term complications of ignoring an undescended testicle, treatment should be considered whenever cryptorchidism is documented after the age of six months. It remains to be confirmed whether early treatment of this condition ameliorates the increase in malignancy and decrease in fertility that is associated with cryptorchidism. Only by early therapy and ongoing studies can the long-term results of our current recommended treatment be assessed.

HYDRONEPHROSIS

Routine use of ultrasonography has led to early diagnosis of hydronephrosis. Nevertheless, careful palpation of the abdomen of a newborn remains the mainstay of diagnosis of abdominal masses, especially those of renal origin. Early diagnosis and urologic referral is important for a positive outcome.

The principal causes of hydronephrosis in infants and children are 1) ureteropelvic junction obstruction; 2) uretero-vesical junction obstruction; 3) reflux; and 4) a dysmorphic urinary tract.

Silent hydronephrosis is sometimes identified in a work-up for congenital malformations, palpable masses, or failure to thrive. More frequently, there are the signs and symptoms associated with urinary tract obstruction, such as fever, pyelonephritis, sepsis, flank pain, and pyuria.

Uretero-pelvic junction obstruction is usually treated by pyeloplasty. Uretero-vesical junction obstruction is relatively rare and results in mega ureter as well as hydronephrosis. The disorder may be mechanical (stenosis) or functional (an aperistaltic segment) in origin. Surgery is the accepted form of treatment.

Reflux is due to congenital malpositioning of the ureteral orifice. Lower grades of reflux tend to resolve spontaneously. Treatment is aimed at keeping the urine sterile while the bladder matures and reflux resolves. If a child is on prophylactic antibiotic treatment, urinalysis and urine culture every three to four months are recommended. In more severe or unresponsive cases of reflux, surgical reimplantation of the ureter is performed. The success rate is greater than 90%. Reflux tends to occur with increased frequency in siblings (30%) and children (60%) of individuals with a history of reflux. Patients falling into these categories should be evaluated.

The dysmorphic urinary system may or may not cause problems. Consequently, it is important to assess renal function to see which of these patients have reflux and which have obstruction and not be guided solely by the radiographic appearance of urinary anatomy. The principal diagnostic modalities used to work up patients with hydronephrosis are ultrasonography, intravenous pyelography, voiding cystourethrogram, and renal scintiscan.

All of the causes of hydronephrosis can vary widely in the degree of dysfunction they produce. Treatment is frequently surgical and success rates are generally good, especially if diagnosis and treatment are accomplished before renal damage ensues.

HYDROCELE

There are three broad categories of hydroceles in the neonate: communicating, noncommunicating, and reactive. A communicating hydrocele is the result of a patent processus vaginalis that creates an open channel between the peritoneum and the tunica vaginalis. This allows for communication of fluid between the scrotum and peritoneum, accounting for both a diurnal variation in scrotal size as well as the characteristic inguinal swelling. A noncommunicating (or simple) hydrocele, which is rare in children, represents a segmental obliteration of the processus vaginalis, leaving a sac of fluid around the testicle, but no communication with the peritoneum. This type of hydrocele does not vary in size. The reactive hydrocele is secondary to infection, trauma, or testicular torsion. It also has no communication with the peritoneum.

The natural history of hydroceles in the first year of life is dynamic. More than one half of the hydroceles disappear secondary to the ongoing obliteration of the processus vaginalis or reabsorption of the noncommunicating hydrocele. It is because of this that many clinicians recommend observation for hydroceles in the first year of life. Indications for early intervention include a communicating hydrocele with marked changes in size. A communicating hydrocele is equivalent to a hernia and should be repaired promptly to preclude incarceration of bowel. Reactive hydroceles resolve spontaneously and do not require separate attention other than treatment for their causative disease.

In general, the surgical approach to scrotal pathology is through the groin. The overwhelming majority of hydroceles that persist after one year of age are of the communicating type. Approaching the hydrocele through the groin allows for identification of the processus vaginalis and its ligation. The actual hydrocele sac that surrounds the testicle does not require resection once it is no longer in continuity with the peritoneum. By reducing the extent of the surgical dissection, the physician can minimize the number of complications. Even when the operation is performed by an experienced surgeon, there are known complications; such complications consist of injury to the vas deferens and testicular artery with subsequent testicular atrophy and decreased fertility. It is for this reason that many surgeons choose not to explore the contralateral groin unless a known hernia or hydrocele exists.

CIRCUMCISION

The surgical procedure most commonly performed on newborn male children in the United States is circumcision. When done by an experienced practitioner, circumcision is a safe procedure. The indications for routine newborn circumcision continue to be debated. The American Academy of Pediatrics in 1989 agreed on the following statement: "Newborn circumcision has potential medical benefits and advantages as well as disadvantages and risks. When circumcision is being considered, the benefits and risks should be explained to the parents and informed consent obtained." Absolute contraindications for circumcision are the presence of hypospadias, epispadias, chordee, or anomalies of the penile skin. Several recent studies have reported a greater frequency of urinary tract infections in uncircumcised infant boys (1.8%) than in those that have been circumcised (0.2%). Generally speaking, the infections were not severe; however, they did require hospitalization and parenteral antibiotics when they occurred in neonates.

The two most common techniques of circumcision in neonates involve use of the Gomco clamp and the Plastibell. Meticulous attention to detail is the best way to ensure a good result and prevent potential disastrous complications. Circumcision begins with an examination of the penis and prepuce. Excess dorsal skin should alert the clinician to the possibility of hypospadias or chordee. The next step is the complete release of the foreskin from the glans, commonly achieved with a small curved hemostat. This allows for definitive identification of the location of the meatus. Whether the Gomco clamp or Plastibell is used, the device must fit properly to protect the glans and ensure excision of the appropriate amount of skin. The amount of skin to be excised should be determined with the skin on the shaft of the penis lying in its natural relaxed state. All penile shaft skin distal to the corona of the glans should be excised. After removal of the device, a vaseline gauze dressing is loosely applied and changed once a day for five days. Reported complications include hemorrhage (1%), infection (0.4%), dehiscence (0.16%), denudation of shaft (0.05%), glandular injury (0.02%), and urinary retention (0.02%).

BALANOPOSTHITIS AND BALANITIS

Balanoposthitis is a fairly common infection of the glans and overlying prepuce (incidence 6%), which usually responds to oral and topical antibiotics and warm baths. The most frequent cause is poor hygiene. If simple treatments are not successful, parenteral antibiotics or circumcision may be required. Most commonly, a mixed flora of organisms are cultured from the exudate. There have been reports of both Group A beta hemolytic *Streptococcus* and Group B *Streptococcus* causing balanitis. In sexually active teenagers, trichomonal balanitis and candidal infections are diagnostic differentials and should prompt investigation of sexual partners. The first episode of balanitis may not be the last, and repeated episodes of balanitis can lead to preputial scarring and phimosis.

Therefore, once an episode of balanitis has occurred, circumcision should be considered as an option for further management.

URINARY TRACT INFECTION

The urinary tract ranks second only to the upper respiratory tract as a source of morbidity from bacterial infection in childhood. The neonatal period is the only time that the male incidence of urinary infection exceeds that of the female. Boys have about a 1% chance of developing an infection during childhood. In newborn boys, the incidence of asymptomatic bacilluria is 1.5%, but it decreases to 0.2% by the time boys are of school age. Incidence of urinary infection is slightly increased in uncircumcised newborn boys. The chance of a girl developing an infection during childhood is close to 3%. Random screening of pre-school and school-age girls shows asymptomatic bacilluria in 1%. The incidence is dependent on age and sex and seems to peak around two years of age, a time that coincides with toilet training, and then returns to a baseline value between 1% and 2%.

The signs and symptoms of urinary tract infection in older child are similar to those seen in the adult population, namely voiding dysfunction, dysuria, hematuria, incontinence, suprapubic or flank tenderness, lethargy, and fever. In neonates, however, the symptoms are much more subtle. Weight loss is most often the prominent symptom, followed by irritability, fever, cyanosis, and disorders of the central nervous system. Thus, nonspecific complaints or problems should raise the suspicion of a urinary tract infection in a newborn but should not lead to hasty conclusions. Fewer than 20% of infants with nonspecific complaints and only 18% of children with specific voiding complaints have a urinary tract infection.

Documentation of infection requires that a specimen be obtained and cultured. Urinalysis may suggest the presence of an infection, but the final determination must rest on bacterial growth on a culture. Of the several ways to collect a specimen from a child, the easiest (once the child has been toilet trained) is the midstream "clean catch" method (see Chapter 1). However, that option is not feasible for children who are not toilet trained. There are three other methods, all of which have advantages and disadvantages. The simplest, but least reliable, is the U-bag. A negative culture from a U-bag is meaningful, but if the culture is positive, it is possible that bacteria from the rectum, skin, or prepuce have contaminated the specimen. Therefore, whenever this method produces positive results, the culture should be repeated with a more accurate method.

The other two procedures are somewhat more involved, but each should provide an uncontaminated aliquot of bladder urine. The first is a percutaneous bladder tap. In neonates and infants, the bladder occupies an intraabdominal position, thereby making the procedure easier than in older persons. Still, the bladder should be full and, preferably, palpable. The second method is urethral catheterization. In small girls, visualization of the urethra may be difficult, but with practice the procedure can be mastered easily. A small feeding tube (5 to 8 French) is most appropriate for catheterization. There should be little risk of urethral trauma or introduction of bacteria into the bladder if routine care and antisepsis are used. Any treatment program should be based on an accurate culture and sensitivity. Consequently, it is imperative that the culture be obtained before antibiotics are started because a single dose of medication can produce false-negative results.

Urinary tract infections are often separated into categories based on the presumed location of the inflammation. Cystitis is a urinary tract infection that has been confined to the bladder, whereas pyelonephritis involves the kidney. Accurate differentiation between the two is difficult; clinical signs and symptoms offer the most meaningful clues. High fever, nausea, vomiting, flank pain, and lethargy are usually associated with acute pyelonephritis, whereas dysuria, frequency of urination, urgency of urination, enuresis, suprapubic pain, and low-grade fever are more common with cystitis, although crossover is common. Renal scintiscan offers an objective alternative to the subjectivity of clinical acumen. However, final determination of the scan's sensitivity is still pending.

Epididymitis is an unusual finding in preadolescent boys. The most common cause of epididymitis is retrograde flow through the prostatic ducts and vas deferens. Its recognition is important because symptoms resemble those of testicular torsion. Treatment of the former is antibiotics and bed rest; for the latter, *prompt surgical exploration is mandatory*. The physical findings (i.e., scrotal erythema, swelling, and pain) may be similar for the both entities. Fever in addition to such laboratory findings as leukocytosis, pyuria, and a positive urine culture suggest a diagnosis of epididymitis. Often, because the diagnosis is questionable, scrotal exploration is performed. Once epididymitis is confirmed in a prepubertal child, an intravenous pyelogram or renal ultrasonography should be considered to identify congenital anomalies. Positive findings, with ureteral and vasal abnormalities predominating, can be expected in more than one-third of children with epididymitis. In these cases, correction of the problem often requires surgery.

Currently, most pediatric urologists recommend that all children with a documented urinary tract infection undergo a uroradiologic evaluation. Generally, studies to evaluate both the bladder (voiding cystourethrogram or, in girls, nuclear cystography) and upper tracts (renal ultrasonography, intravenous pyelogram, or renal scintiscan) are suggested. For older girls with simple cystitis, it can be argued that performance of an upper urinary tract study is sufficient because it will reveal any significant pathology. The yield for these evaluations depends on age and sex and ranges up to 50% in young girls with pyelonephritis (primarily from discovery of vesicoureteral reflux). Discovery of an anatomic anomaly, such as obstruction or reflux, must be addressed and prompt referral to a specialist is recommended. Still, most urinary tract infections can be treated adequately on an outpatient basis with a 7- to 10-day course of antibiotics. Shorter courses may be used but are associated with a higher recurrence rate. Occasionally, a child with severe symptoms of pyelonephritis will require hospitalization for parenteral antibiotics and control of nausea. For children with frequently recurring infections (at least four a year), a long-term, low-dose daily prophylactic antibiotic (usually nitrofurantoin or trimethoprim-sulfamethoxazole at one-fourth to one-half of the therapeutic dose) is appropriate. The medications are usually given for 9 to 12 months. Subsequent follow-up should include regular urinalysis and cultures when indicated.

TESTICULAR TORSION

Disorders of the scrotum can range from a benign bug bite to the scrotal wall or significant testicular torsion requiring immediate surgical repair. Torsion of the testicle is one of the few true emergencies in pediatric urology. It is a common intrascrotal disorder in boys and requires prompt surgical intervention to avoid testicular necrosis. Testicular torsion must be differentiated from epididymitis and torsion of a testicular appendage because neither of these conditions requires surgery.

Testicular torsion occurs within the tunica albuginea (intravaginal) or includes the tunica albuginea (extravaginal). Intravaginal torsion is more common and occurs most frequently in early adolescence. It is thought to result from the absence of posterior attachments between the tunica vaginalis and testicle, as such attachments normally stabilize the gonad within the scrotum. Signs of testicular torsion consist of acute onset of severe hemiscrotal pain, nausea, and vomiting. The attacks may be intermittent. Examination reveals an enlarged tender testicle and frequently some degree of scrotal edema. The opposite testicle may be lying in an unusually lateral position. As time progresses, intrascrotal elements become confluent and torsion may be difficult to differentiate from acute or chronic epididymitis. Other beneficial studies may include a nuclear technetium scan of the testicles or Doppler ultrasonography of the scrotum to assess testicular blood flow. Prompt surgical exploration and detorsion is mandatory, as irreversible changes in the testicle may occur within four hours. If treatment is not prompt, orchiectomy may be required. Because the abnormality (absence of posterior testicular attachment) is often bilateral, a contralateral scrotal orchiopexy should be done whenever intravaginal torsion is diagnosed.

Extravaginal torsion (torsion of the entire spermatic cord and testicles outside of the tunica vaginalis) occurs almost exclusively in neonates and often occurs before birth. The cause of this disorder may be the absence of adhesions between the scrotum and testicular membranes. It usually presents as a small, hard, nontender mass replacing the testicle in a discolored hemiscrotum. Treatment is controversial (even prompt surgical exploration reveals a necrotic testicle) and orchiectomy is almost universally accepted as the appropriate treatment. Although evidence is lacking to show that the defect is bilateral, surgeons often correct the contralateral testicle because subsequent torsion could have devastating results.

Torsion of a testicular appendage must be distinguished from testicular torsion. Unless the diagnosis can be made with confidence, the practitioner is obligated to pursue a more thorough evaluation or surgically explore the acute scrotum. The symptoms of torsion of a testicular appendage are less severe than those of testicular torsion. At times, the appendage is palpable in the upper aspect of the scrotum, and, if infarcted, a pathognomonic blue dot may be visible. Appropriate treatment consists of bed rest; the natural course is slow, steady improvement.

Suggested Reading

Barthold JS: Cryptorchidism, in Walsh PC and others (eds): *Campbell's Urology*, ed 6, Philadelphia, WB Saunders, 1994.

Hadziselimovic F: *Cryptorchidism: Management and Implications*, Berlin, Springer-Verlag, 1983.

Kogan SJ: Cryptorchidism, in Kalalis PP, King LR, Belman AB (eds): *Clinical Pediatric Urology*, ed 2, vol 2, Philadelphia, WB Saunders, 1985, pp 864–887.

Rozanski TA, Bloom DA: The undescended testis: theory and management, *Urol Clin North Am* 22(1):107–118, 1995.

11

Emergency Urology

Urologic emergencies, either real or perceived, are relatively common. Many common urologic problems may present as true emergencies. These include urinary retention, renal or ureteral colic, urosepsis, gross hematuria, extreme dysuria (which has also been characterized as stranguria), testicular pain, and such penile problems as priapism. Appropriate prompt recognition and definitive management of these conditions will quite often reduce associated morbidity and increase long-term success of treatment.

URINARY RETENTION

Urinary retention, defined as the inability to evacuate the full bladder, commonly presents as an emergency. Urinary retention is caused by detrusor failure or, more commonly, by urinary outlet obstruction. Regardless of the etiology, this condition can have deleterious effects on the bladder and upper urinary tract as well as the overall electrolyte status.

Manifestations

Although urinary retention is characterized by an inability to empty the full bladder, patients may or may not perceive bladder fullness. Chronic urinary retention, which is common in patients with neurogenic vesical dysfunction and prostatism, may be characterized by dribbling incontinence. The incontinence may occur both day and night. Patients typically have no awareness of bladder distention, although some patients with chronic retention may complain of urinary frequency and nocturia. In rare cases, the only symptoms may be an increased abdominal girth. Patients with acute urinary retention typically perceive bladder distention and bladder discomfort. Problems that commonly lead to urinary retention are listed in Table 11–1. Populations at risk typically have a characteristic history. For example, men older than 60 years of age are at significant risk of retention because of prostatism. Patients with neurologic-based voiding difficulties typically have a history of neurologic problems, perhaps even a specific diagnosis, such as spinal cord injury. Younger, middle-aged men may give a history of gonococcal urethritis and/or voiding difficulties as youths. Patients who have previously undergone a prostatectomy may develop urethral strictures and/or bladder neck contractures that may cause acute urinary retention. Similarly, patients taking anticholinergic drugs for other reasons (e.g., irritative bowel syndrome), are certainly at risk for pharmacologically induced retention.

Diagnosis

The diagnosis of urinary retention can ordinarily be revealed by physical examination. The bladder usually is palpable above the pubic symphysis and may extend 1

TABLE 11–1.

Common Etiologies of Urinary Retention

Obstructive Etiologies	Primary Detrusor Insufficiency
Urethral stricture	Detrusor areflexia
Enlarged prostate	Multiple sclerosis
Lower genitourinary tract malignancy	Iatrogenic injury during abdominal or back surgery
Pelvic malignancy	
Bladder stones	Spinal cord injury
Foreign body	Myelomeningocele
Blood clot	
Posterior urethral valves	
Ureterocele	

or 2 centimeters above the symphysis or to the umbilicus. A postvoid abdominal ultrasonographic examination or determination of the postvoid catheterized urinary residual measurement is typically diagnostic. The elevated bladder dome may be percussed as it rises above the symphysis. A urine volume of more than 200 cc after attempted micturition is characteristic of inefficient bladder emptying.

Management

Management is determined by the underlying cause of retention. Men with uncomplicated prostatism can usually be catheterized with a 16-French standard Foley-type urethral catheter. If such a catheter cannot be passed atraumatically, then the problem is more likely to be urethral stricture or bladder neck contracture.

A coude-tipped urethral catheter (Fig. 11–1) is the instrument of choice for catheterizing patients with extremely enlarged prostate glands and/or patients with a high probability of bladder neck contractures. The coude tip passes over median bar prostatic enlargements with greater ease and less trauma than does the standard-tipped catheter. While a routine catheter can be passed by the primary-care physician, further instrumentation usually demands the expertise of the specialist.

Filiforms and followers are the catheters of choice if a tight meatal stenosis or urethral stricture is present. These catheters should be passed very gently by an experienced individual. They may be extremely traumatic and damaging to the urethra if used incorrectly. After successful passage of a filiform, the smallest caliber hollow follower available is attached to the filiform and is gently inserted with lubrication into the urinary bladder to effect drainage. Typically, the

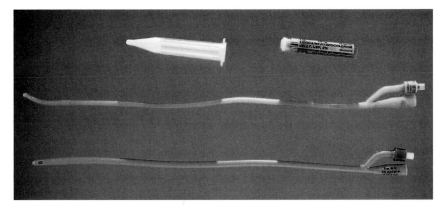

FIG. 11–1.

A standard-tip Foley catheter, a coudé tip Foley catheter, and lidocaine jelly with the catheter syringe used for insertion.

follower is left indwelling for 24 hours to soften the stricture. Afterward, the stricture can be further dilated on an elective basis to accept a larger catheter.

A suprapubic punch cystotomy is probably a more effective emergency treatment for most primary-care physicians than is the use of filiforms and followers. The punch cystostomy technique is appropriate when physical examination or ultrasonography show the bladder to be distended and use of the standard or coude-tipped urethral catheters is not successful.

Techniques

Urethral Catheterization

In both men and women, the urethra should be well lubricated with anesthetic jelly. Lidocaine-impregnated, water-soluble jelly is readily available in most clinics and emergency rooms. Ten to 20 milliliters of anesthetic jelly should be instilled into the urethra using a catheter-tipped syringe. After the catheter syringe is lightly inserted into the urethral meatus, the entire urethra is slowly filled with the anesthetic jelly. In men, the glans penis should be grasped with the nondominant hand and extended away from the pubis in the erect position (Fig. 11–2). The urethral catheter is then inserted with the dominant hand. Some resistance is usually encountered at the external urethral sphincter. Slow sustained pressure in this area coupled with deep breaths by the patient with the mouth open will usually aid in relaxation of the sphincter and easy passage of the catheter.

When available, a coude-tipped catheter should be chosen over a standard-tipped catheter. The catheter is secured by inflating the balloon with 5 cc of water and withdrawing the catheter until the balloon "hangs" at the bladder neck. The catheter should be attached to gravity drainage, and 24-hour urine output should be monitored.

Unsuccessful catheter replacement should not be followed by more aggressive attempts. Use of a catheter guide in an attempt to stiffen the Foley catheter and forcibly pass it beyond the obstruction should be avoided. Such measures invariably cause urethral trauma, which may lead to secondary strictures, urosepsis, or other problems.

Suprapubic Punch Cystostomy

Diagnosis of urinary retention should be confirmed prior to placement of a punch cystostomy. Confirmation is achieved by infiltrating the abdominal wall and skin two centimeters above the pubic synthesis with a 1% lidocaine solution. Thereafter, a 22-gauge needle attached to a 10-cc syringe is inserted through the anesthetized skin into the distended urinary bladder. Aspiration of the plunger should yield an easy flow of obvious urine. After this confirmation, the 22-gauge needle is removed and trocar-assisted cystostomy is performed.

Special trocar punch cystostomy kits are commercially available (Fig. 11–3). Most emergency rooms have an inventory of such kits. Alternatively, a 14-gauge intravenous needle and a pediatric 5-French feeding tube may also be used. The large-caliber needle is inserted through anesthetized skin into the urinary bladder. As urine flows through the needle, the 5-French pediatric feeding tube or an intravenous cannula is threaded through the needle into the urinary

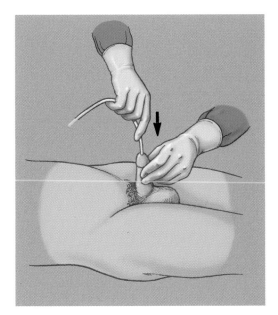

FIG. 11–2.

Extension of penis for catheter insertion. This position prevents urethral trauma at the peno-scrotal junction during catheter placement.

bladder. Thereafter, the needle is removed from the abdominal wall and the catheter is secured to the skin with a silk suture.

Occasionally, patients will present with urinary retention secondary to blood clots within the bladder. Predisposing conditions are listed in Table 11–2. Quite often, the clot-containing bladder is palpably distended on abdominal examination. Placement of a Foley catheter into the bladder reveals gross hema-

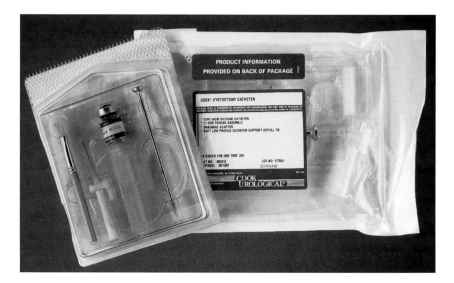

FIG. 11–3.

Commercially available suprapubic cystostomy sets.

TABLE 11–2.

Common Etiologies
of Clot Retention

Recent genitourinary surgery

Genitourinary malignancy

Abdominal/perineal radiotherapy

Trauma

Chemotherapy (e.g., Cytoxan®
   [Bristol-Myers Squibb])

Bleeding diathesis

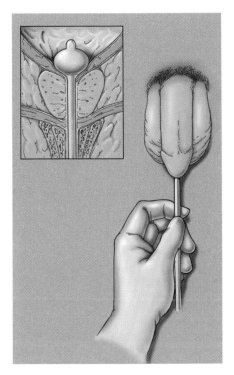

FIG. 11–4.

Catheter traction with an inflated intravesical balloon.

turia with clots. Incomplete emptying of the bladder due to use of an average but small-diameter catheter is commonly encountered.

Adequate evacuation of the bladder in a patient with clot retention requires a large Foley catheter (22 French or larger). Manual irrigation with a 60-cc piston syringe and normal saline should be used to evacuate clots. If a clear effluent cannot be obtained with manual irrigation, continuous irrigation utilizing a three-way Foley catheter may be necessary. Quite commonly, urologic referral is helpful. All clots should be evacuated from the bladder prior to initiating three-way irrigation. Catheter traction with an inflated intravesical balloon is often helpful if the bleeding is from the bladder neck or prostatic bed (Fig. 11–4). One caveat to the use of manual irrigation of the bladder in clot retention is that if the patient has had recent open bladder surgery, aggressive manual irrigation may result in bladder rupture.

After establishment of adequate bladder drainage, the patient's urine output must be carefully monitored.

Acute urinary retention does not usually warrant overnight hospitalization. However, chronic urinary retention that is typically characterized by elevations in blood urea nitrogen and creatinine may result in postobstructive diuresis. Thus, patients with chronic retention are candidates for overnight (24-hour) observation. In patients with chronic urinary retention, nephrogenic diabetes insipidus may develop. Volume as well as potassium replacement is usually necessary in a closely monitored setting if this diagnosis is strongly suspected.

Once relief of the urinary obstruction is achieved, the etiology of the condition must be determined. Imaging studies, including retrograde urethrography, voiding cystourethrography, and intravenous pyelography, are often helpful in making the correct diagnosis. Cystourethroscopy and urodynamics are also beneficial in selected patients—the former to visualize the exact nature of the obstruction and the latter to precisely document the type of bladder failure. Urodynamics should be postponed until the overstretched bladder has had sufficient time to regain baseline tone. This usually takes three to four days and may take weeks if the bladder obstruction has been long term.

RENAL OR URETERAL COLIC

Excruciating flank, loin, or lower quadrant abdominal pain of abrupt onset is characteristic of renal or ureteral colic. The severity of the pain and its abrupt onset typically trigger immediate emergency phone calls and emergency room visits. Primary initiatives are directed toward establishing the diagnosis and relieving pain. Emergency treatment to remove the obstructing stone is rarely indicated.

Manifestations

Depending on the point of ureteral irritation, all or part of the dermatome that shares innervation with the ureter may be affected (Fig. 11–5). The pain tends to be sharp and intermittent in quality. If ureteral obstruction or irritation becomes long-standing, the pain experienced by the patient may lessen without improvement in the underlying pathology. If distal ureteral irritation is present, irritative bladder symptoms characterized by urinary frequency may be experienced.

The most common etiology of ureteral colic is nephrolithiasis. Classically, patients will present with severe pain out of proportion to findings on physical examination. Great care must be used in making the presumptive diagnosis of ureteral colic, because many other intraabdominal disease states may have similar symptoms and findings (Table 11–3).

Diagnosis

Urinalysis usually reveals the presence of hematuria, although its absence does not rule out the diagnosis of ureteral colic. Pyuria and bacteriuria may also be noted on urine evaluation. In patients suspected of having ureteral colic, upper tract imaging is necessary. If the patient has a serum creatinine of less than 2.0 and is not allergic to intravenous contrast, intravenous pyelography is preferred. This technique will show the anatomy of the upper tracts, the presence or absence of stones, and the degree of ureteral obstruction (Fig. 11–6), if present. Alternatively, x-rays of the kidney, ureter, and bladder as well as renal ultrasonography may be obtained. This combination of imaging studies gives the clinician information about upper tract

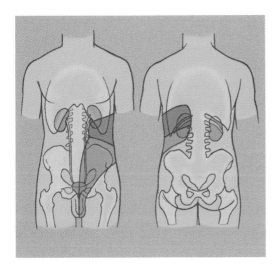

FIG. 11–5.

Dermatome of area to which ureteral irritation may be referred.

TABLE 11–3.

Diagnostic Differentials of Renal or Ureteral Colic

Acute cholecystitis, acute cholelithiasis

Acute appendicitis

Pelvic inflammatory disease

Diverticulosis and/or diverticulitis

Intestinal obstruction

Leaking abdominal aortic aneurysm

Musculoskeletal sprains

Herniated nucleus pulposus

Herpes zoster (shingles)

Gastrointestinal dysfunction with ileus and/or toxic colonic dilatation anatomy, the presence or absence of hydronephrosis, and stones, but it gives incomplete information about the degree of obstruction, if present.

Management

Patients with a presumptive diagnosis of ureteral colic should be given intravenous hydration and intravenous analgesia if an acute abdominal process has been ruled out. If radiologic imaging confirms the presence of a small (<5 mm), partially obstructing distal ureteral stone, conservative management is an option. Patients should be instructed to stay well hydrated, take oral analgesics as needed for pain, and strain their urine. Any passed stones should be kept for analysis. Urologic follow-up should be arranged prior to patient discharge.

Indications for immediate treatment of ureteral colic are listed in Table 11–4. In most cases, the obstructed upper tract should be drained by placement of a retrograde ureteral stent or by performance of percutaneous nephrostomy. After the patient is stabilized, the obstructive stone may be removed electively by lithotripsy, endourologic devices, or a combination of these modalities. Currently,

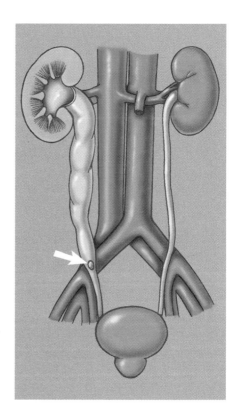

FIG. 11–6.

Drawing showing an obstructing stone. (From Tanagho EA, McAninch JW: *Smith's General Urology,* ed 3, Norwalk, CN, Appleton & Lange, 1992, p 171. Reproduced with permission.)

TABLE 11–4.

Indications for Immediate Treatment of Ureteral Colic

Stone in one kidney

Urinary tract infection with fever

High-grade obstruction

Large proximal ureteral stones

Stone impaction

Severe symptoms (unresponsive nausea, vomiting, pain)

some patients are managed with acute intervention (lithotripsy or ureteroscopy) prior to drainage of the affected urinary tract. However, candidates for such manipulation must be carefully chosen to avoid increasing patient morbidity.

UROSEPSIS

Urinary tract infection may lead to systemic sepsis. Significant morbidity and mortality can be associated with such sepsis.

Manifestations

The patient usually presents with abrupt onset of high fever. Symptoms of pain or dysuria may point to the kidney, bladder, prostate gland, or urethra as the principally involved organ. Bacteriuria usually is present. In advanced cases, the patient may appear pale, weak, and debilitated. Such patients may be on the border of hypovolemic endotoxic shock.

Diagnosis

The medical history and physical findings usually indicate a diagnosis of urosepsis. Intravenous pyelography, urinalysis, and urine culture should also point toward the diagnosis. When possible, renal tomograms both with and without contrast should be made during the urogram. These studies may reveal the presence of small, poorly opaque obstructing stones and/or the presence of a renal cortical mass (carbuncle or perinephric abscess). Bilateral renal ultrasonography (Fig. 11–7) is nearly equivalent to a contrast urogram in evaluating upper

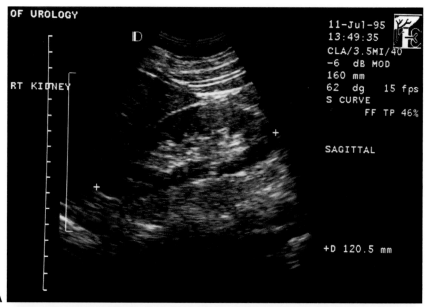

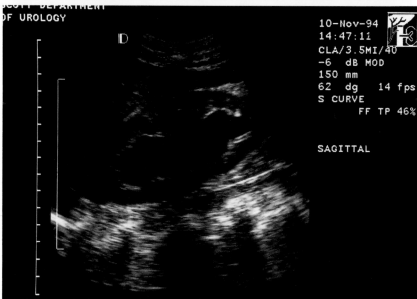

FIG. 11–7.

A, Normal sonogram. **B,** Sonogram demonstrating hydronephrosis.

tract obstruction. Hydronephrosis and the presence of symptomatic bacteriuria establish the diagnosis of pending or overt urosepsis.

Predisposing factors to urosepsis include increasing patient age, immediate prior instrumentation of the urinary tract, urinary tract obstruction, and preexisting bacteriuria (Table 11–5). In patients with grossly infected urine, the etiology of their systemic sepsis may be evident. In other patients, the relationship between clinical sepsis and the urinary tract may be difficult to determine. In patients with sepsis of unknown etiology, bladder catheterization should be performed—not only for adequate urinary drainage but also to monitor urinary output.

If bacteriuria or pyuria is present, the upper tracts should be imaged radiologically to rule out upper tract obstruction, perinephric abscess, or other upper tract pathology that could predispose the patient to sepsis. Currently, abdominal-pelvic computed tomography is the radiologic modality of choice for these studies. Computed tomography should be done with a Foley catheter in place to rule out a lower urinary tract etiology to upper tract dilation. Another clue to a diagnosis of urosepsis is a positive blood culture for typical urologic pathogens. If blood cultures are positive for uropathogens and the etiology of a patient's sepsis has not been ascertained, reexamination of the urinary tract is indicated.

Management

Blood and urine specimens should be submitted for aerobic and anaerobic cultures after which systemic parenteral antimicrobials should be administered. Ampicillin and gentamicin are good first-line choices in the absence of a history of antibiotic use and/or known bacterial sensitivities. Analgesics should be

TABLE 11–5.
Common Causes of Urosepsis

Obstructing ureteral stone with pyonephrosis
Staghorn calculus with urinary infection
Ureteral obstruction with proximal urinary tract infection
Urinary retention with urinary infection
Acute prostatitis with prostatic abscess
Perinephric abscess or renal carbuncle
Urethral stricture with periurethral abscess
Fournier's gangrene
Foreign body within urinary tract (e.g., Foley catheter)

administered to control pain after which prompt relief of urinary obstruction is warranted. Relief of urinary obstruction can be achieved via the retrograde route (cystoscopy and retrograde catheterization with or without ureteral stents) or by antegrade techniques (percutaneous nephrostomy and insertion of universal ureteral stent). Such procedures are typically warranted immediately after the diagnosis is made. In certain cases, 12 hours of antimicrobial therapy may be administered prior to surgical relief of obstructive uropathy. However, surgery should not be delayed because of fears of hypovolemic shock. In the face of urinary tract obstruction, the presence of impending hypovolemic shock is an absolute indication for surgical intervention.

Perinephric abscesses, renal cortical abscesses (carbuncles), prostatic abscesses, and periurethral abscesses may contribute to or establish urosepsis in the absence of overt urinary tract obstruction. However, even these conditions may be associated with ureteral or urethral obstruction. Drainage of the abscesses may not be warranted until after a few hours of systemic antimicrobial treatment. However, it is incumbent upon the attending physician to exclude obstructive uropathy with the initial evaluation. Thus, use of ultrasonography or urethral catheters or suprapubic punctures may be warranted.

Definitive treatment generally can be delayed until the acute uroseptic condition has been adequately remedied. When the patient is afebrile and physiologically sound, definitive treatment of the primary underlying problem can be undertaken on an elective basis.

GROSS HEMATURIA

Gross hematuria is a manifestation of some underlying disease. The disorder in the absence of significant symptoms is not a true emergency; however, it commonly alarms the patient to such an agitated state that emergency evaluation and treatment are sought. The magnitude, frequency, and duration of hematuria do not forecast its severity. A soothing explanation may be sufficient early treatment to calm the "unnerved" patient.

Manifestations

In men, gross hematuria may be initial, terminal, or total. Initial hematuria (when only the first few milliliters of the urinary stream contain blood) suggest urethral disease. Terminal hematuria suggests prostatic disease. Total hematuria suggests that the entire bladder volume is contaminated with blood and thus implies upper tract disease.

Hematuria may be symptomatic or asymptomatic. Symptomatic hematuria is hematuria in the presence of pain, dysuria, fever, or other sequelae of urinary pathology. Asymptomatic microscopic hematuria, however, may be the first sign

TABLE 11–6.

Common Causes of Hematuria

Hematuria may arise from renal, ureteral, vesical, prostatic, or urethral abnormalities. The following abnormalities may cause hematuria:

- Malignant tumors
- Benign tumors
- Cysts
- Stones
- Trauma (even jogging)
- Infection
- Instrumentation
- Intrinsic (internal) obstruction
- Extrinsic (external or nonluminal) compressive obstruction
- Anomalies, such as hemoglobinuria or sickle trait disease

of a significant underlying urologic problem. It deserves thorough, but elective, evaluation. Potential sources of hematuria are detailed in Table 11–6.

Diagnosis

The etiology of gross hematuria is typically established with intravenous urography and endoscopy. Intravenous pyelography and office cystoscopy with a flexible cystoscope are usually sufficient to establish the underlying cause of hematuria. In selected cases, more rigorous imaging consisting of computed tomography, magnetic resonance imaging, and angiography are warranted. However, these advanced tests are rarely warranted in the initial evaluation. Only if the initial evaluation demonstrates a complex renal or extraperitoneal mass are the advanced studies warranted. For the simple evaluation of gross hematuria, intravenous urography and cystoscopy are usually sufficient.

Management

Management of hematuria requires management of the underlying etiologic condition. In some cases, no major pathology can be identified as the source of the hematuria. If proteinuria is present or if there is a history of diabetes mellitus, nephrologic evaluation and possible renal biopsy are serious considerations. However, in the absence of hypertension, proteinuria, azotemia, or obvious uropathologic conditions, extensive nephrologic evaluation usually is unwarranted.

DYSURIA AND STRANGURY

Dysuria is painful or difficult urination. Strangury is slow, painful urination due to spasms of the urethra or the bladder. Strangury is an advanced form of dysuria.

Manifestations

Inflammatory conditions of the bladder, urethra, vulva, and prostate gland typically underlie dysuria and strangury. Urethritis with bacteria, viruses, ureaplasma, or protozoan organisms most typically cause the symptoms. Noninfectious urethritis may occur as a consequence of trauma in both men and women. Aggressive sexual foreplay, excessive masturbation, or foreign bodies have been implicated in noninfectious urethritis. In men, the reflux of sterile urine into the ejaculatory ducts, prostate gland, vas deferens, and epididymis may occur as a consequence of heavy lifting or straining. These conditions may also create noninfectious urethritis, prostatitis, and epididymitis, all of which lead to dysuria and strangury.

Urinary stones in the bladder, urethra, and distal ureter may also produce these symptoms, as may benign and malignant tumors of the bladder, urethra, and prostate gland. Typically, the underlying pathology contributes to urinary infection, which leads to the symptoms. Neuromuscular conditions, such as diabetes and demyelinating neurologic diseases, may also contribute to the symptom complex. Thus, evaluation and treatment of the symptoms should also be accompanied by complete evaluation of the urologic system to look for underlying pathologic conditions.

Management

Management focuses on relieving the symptoms and evaluating the urologic system for underlying pathology. Urinalysis and urine culture might be initiated at the initial visit. The finding of white blood cells and bacteria in urinary sediment is sufficient to establish a diagnosis of urinary infection. Treatment may be initiated with broad-spectrum antimicrobials (e.g., quinolones) and with urinary sedatives, such as Pyridium® (Parke-Davis). Also, anticholinergic medications may be of value in minimizing bladder and urethral spasm. Oxybutynin, Banthine® (Roberts), and Pro-Banthine® (Roberts) are useful in this regard.

After initial treatment, elective evaluation is appropriate. Such evaluation should consist of imaging studies of the upper urinary tract followed by cystoscopy. Other more advanced diagnostic techniques are rarely indicated if the history and physical examination and basic evaluations do not demonstrate significant underlying urologic pathology.

TESTICULAR TORSION

Acute scrotal pain is a common complaint in preadolescents, adolescents, and young adults but can be seen in men of all ages. Diagnostic differentials are listed in Table 11–7. Testicular torsion can have dire consequences; thus, this complaint must always be considered an emergency.

Manifestations

Patients with testicular torsion classically present with acute pain that is constant and severe. Abdominal pain as well as nausea and vomiting often coincide with onset of these symptoms. Neonatal torsion is most commonly noted as a painless enlarged hemiscrotum during the infant's initial physical examination. Scrotal erythema or discoloration and a hydrocele are also commonly seen.

Diagnosis

A careful history is essential. A history of recent scrotal trauma, dysuria, hematuria, urethral discharge, sexual activity, and length of time since onset of symptoms should be noted.

Physical examination should include abdominal, genital, and digital rectal examinations. Particular attention should be paid to the presence or absence of urethral discharge, the position or axis of the affected testicle (Fig. 11–8), the presence or absence of an ipsilateral hydrocele, testicular or epi-

---

TABLE 11–7.

Possible Etiologies of Acute Disorders of the Scrotum

Testicular torsion

Epididymitis or orchitis

Torsion of testicular appendage

Trauma with or without testicular rupture

Testicular malignancy

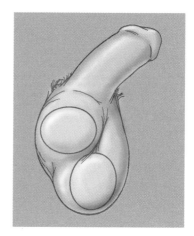

FIG. 11–8.

Transverse position of testicle as seen in testicular torsion.

didymal induration or mass, or scrotal discoloration. Urinalysis should be obtained to check for evidence of infection.

Diagnostic imaging often aids the clinician in making the correct diagnosis. Doppler ultrasonography shows epididymal and testicular architecture quite well and, in experienced hands, can demonstrate the presence or absence of blood flow to the testicle. The technetium radioisotope scrotal scan may also be helpful in differentiating testicular torsion from epididymitis or orchitis by evaluating blood flow to the affected hemiscrotum and comparing it with flow to the unaffected side. A marked reduction in blood flow is evidence of testicular torsion.

Management

If diagnostic imaging cannot be immediately obtained or is equivocal, scrotal exploration should be performed. In cases of testicular torsion, salvage rates of the testicle hinge on the duration of ischemia. Therefore, scrotal exploration should be performed as soon as possible if a diagnosis of testicular torsion is a possibility. It is far better to explore the scrotum and find acute epididymitis than to lose a testicle because of a prolonged work-up with delayed surgery. If testicular torsion is found during scrotal exploration, orchiopexy is performed if the affected testicle is viable or orchiectomy is done if it is nonviable. Orchiopexy is then completed on the contralateral side to prevent future torsion of the remaining testicle.

PRIAPISM

Priapism is a painful condition. It is characterized by prolonged erection that is not associated with sexual stimulation.

Manifestations

Priapism may be of idiopathic origin or secondary to other conditions. Table 11–8 lists possible etiologies of priapism. Priapism is most commonly is caused by a veno-occlusive disorder of penile drainage (low-flow) or is, less commonly, secondary to high arterial inflow.

Diagnosis

The distinction between high-flow priapism and veno-occlusive priapism can be made by penile corporeal blood gas determinations or Doppler ultrasonography. Veno-occlusive (low-flow) priapism is characterized by hypoxia, acidosis, and poor arterial inflow. High-flow priapism is characterized by normal arterial oxygen concentration, normal pH, and good arterial inflow.

Management

Treatment of low-flow priapism must be initiated quickly in order to prevent hypoxic injury to the tissues of the penis. The long-term success of intervention becomes markedly lower if detumescence is not achieved in 48 to 72 hours after the onset of symptoms. In sickle cell disease, initial therapy consists of hydration, alkalinization, analgesics, and hypertransfusion in order to lower the percentage of abnormal hemoglobin S remaining in the patient. In patients with non-sickle cell disease, low-flow priapism, or with sickle cell disease refractory to medical therapy, injection of a weak solution of an alpha agonist into the corpora cavernosa (Table 11–9) often results in detumescence. Other therapies include corporeal irrigation with saline or alpha agonist solution and use of various corporeal shunts (Table 11–10), if conservative therapy fails. Consultation with a specialist may be helpful if these invasive procedures are indicated.

TABLE 11–8.
Possible Etiologies of Priapism

Idiopathic
Thromboembolic phenomenon (sickle cell anemia, leukemia)
Malignant penile infiltration
Traumatic (perineal, genital)
Medication and chemicals (alcohol, cocaine, psychotropic agents, antihypertensives)
Intracavernous injection (papaverine, phentolamine, prostaglandin E_1)

TABLE 11–9.

Alpha Agonists Used for Priapism

Drugs	Dose
Epinephrine	10 to 20 μg
Phenylephrine	100 to 500 μg
Ephedrine	50 to 100 mg
Norepinephrine	10 to 20 μg

Agents should be administered directly into the corpora cavernosa via percutaneous injection. This may be repeated every 5 minutes or until detumescence occurs. Maximum administration is 3 doses.

TABLE 11–10.

Shunts for Priapism

Corpora cavernosa/corpus spongiosum

Corpora cavernosa/saphenous vein

Corpora cavernosa/glans penis

If high-flow priapism is suggested by blood gas or Doppler ultrasonography, arteriography is indicated. If an arteriovenous fistula is documented, it may be treated by embolization or may be surgically ligated.

FORESKIN PROBLEMS

Phimosis is a condition in which the foreskin cannot be retracted over the glans penis. In young children, this condition is not pathologic unless inflammation, infection, or ballooning of the foreskin is noted. The foreskin should be easily retractable in children older than five years of age and in adults. In patients with phimosis, it is difficult to maintain good hygiene and the patient is predisposed to balanitis and penile carcinoma. Treatment is circumcision.

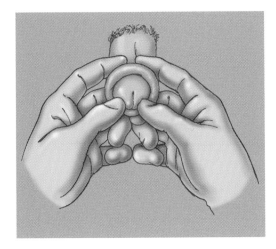

FIG. 11–9.

Manual reduction
of paraphimosis.

Paraphimosis is a condition in which the foreskin is retracted and swelling of the glans penis develops. Treatment must be immediate, as ischemia of the glans can result if the disorder is left untreated. Treatment is manual reduction of the paraphimosis (Fig. 11–9) or a dorsal slit of the foreskin.

CONCLUSION

In summary, most urologic emergencies can be handled by treating the symptoms. The medical history and physical examination, coupled with simple laboratory measures, such as urinalysis, usually point to the underlying problem. Additional studies, such as urine culture or an intravenous urogram, may be arranged on an urgent or elective basis while therapeutic intervention to control the acute symptoms are undertaken. After relief of symptoms, a more complete urologic assessment is appropriate on an elective basis.

INDEX

Note that page numbers followed by "f" designate figures while those followed by "t" designate tables.

A

Abdominal bruit, 41
Abdominal mass, 16–18
Abdominal obesity, and erectile dysfunction, 103
Abdominal pain, 16–18, 142
Abdominal trauma, 36, 40
Abscess(es), prostatic, 10, 80
Acquired cystic disease of kidneys, 40
Acrolein, 35
AIDS, prostatis abscess in, 80
Alcohol abuse, and erectile dysfunction, 102
Alkylating agents, 110
Alpha-adrenergic agonists, for incontinence, 63, 63t
Alpha-adrenergic antagonists
    in benign prostatic hyperplasia, 76
    in impotence, 104
    in prostatodynia, 82
Alpha$_1$-antichymotrypsin, 89
5-Alpha-reductase inhibitors, 76
Alport's syndrome, 35, 36
American Urological Association Symptom Index, 74, 75f
Amphetamines, 104
Anal sphincter, testing of, 58
Anal tone, 10
Androgen replacement, for micropenis, 23
Androgens, inhibition of, 112
Angiography, renal, 41, 42
Angiokeratomas, scrotal, 5
Aniline dyes, 35
Anorchism, 121, 122f, 123
Anthocyanins, 32
Antibiotic prophylaxis, in children, 52, 53, 132
Antibiotic therapy, in female urinary tract infection, 47–50
    in male urinary tract infection, 50–52, 51f
    in prostatitis, 80–82
    in urosepsis, 147, 148
Anticholinergic drugs, 136, 150
Anticoagulants, and hematuria, 35
Antidepressant agents, and erectile dysfunction, 103
Antifungal medications, 5
Antihypertensive agents, and erectile dysfunction, 103
Antiinflammatory agents, and hematuria, 35
Antistreptolysin O titer, 35
Aphrodisiacs, 104
Apomorphine, 104
Arteriovenous fistula, renal, 41, 42
Aspermia, 111

Atherosclerosis, and erectile dysfunction, 101, 103
Atrophic vaginitis, 58
Atrophied testicles, 5f, 18, 22, 121, 122f, 123, 128
Auscultation, in scrotal enlargement, 6
Azoospermia, 111, 116

B

Bacilluria, asymptomatic, 130
Back pain, 16, 18
Bacteria, in urine, 10, 12t
Bacteria, fecal, and urinary tract infection, 46–49
Bacterial cystitis, pyuria in, 31
Bacterial infection, of penis, 23, 129
    of prostate, 77–83, 78t, 79f
Bacteriuria, in colic, 142
    in men, 50
    in pregnancy, 49
    in prostatitis, 81
    relapsing, 81
    in urinary tract infection, 46, 47
    in urosepsis, 145, 147
Balanitis, 23, 154
Balanitis xerotica obliterans, 23
Balanoposthitis, 154
Balloon, intravesical, 141, 141f
Barbotage bladder washings, 42
BCG therapy, intravesical, 82
Benign prostatic hyperplasia, 73–76, 75f
Benzidine, 35
Berger's disease, 34
Bilirubin, in urine, 10, 12t
Biofeedback techniques, in incontinence, 62
Biopsy, of prostate, 87, 91
Bladder, clots in, 140, 140t, 141
    distended, 2
    herniation of, 59
    incomplete emptying of, 20, 21, 137
    neurogenic, 20, 21
    uninhibited, 21, 61, 61f
Bladder cancer, BCG therapy for, 82
    hematuria in, 34, 41
Bladder capacity, 62
Bladder contractions, cough and, 59
    involuntary, 61, 61f
Bladder fullness, in urinary retention, 136
Bladder instability, and incontinence, 59
    and irritative voiding, 21
Bladder outlet obstruction, and acute prostatitis, 80